The Ultimate Tea Recipe Book

Experience the Healing Power and Flavorful Delights of Herbal Teas, Journey Through a Collection of Flavorful and Healing Herbal Tea Recipes, An Essential Herbal TeaBook

Prof. ROSEMARY PURSELL &
B.Sc. JJ GLADSTAR

© Copyright 2024 - All rights reserved.

By reading this document, the reader agrees that under no circumstances is the author responsible for any losses, direct or indirect, which are incurred as a result of the use of information contained within this document, including, but not limited to, — errors, omissions, or inaccuracies.

Table of Content

Introduction

Grab a cozy blanket, put the kettle on, and get ready to dive into the wonderful world of herbal teas! Tea drinking is one of life's simple pleasures that has been practiced for thousands of years. While black and green teas reign supreme, herbal teas offer a flavorful and therapeutic alternative. These caffeine-free infusions are made from dried leaves, seeds, roots, flowers, fruits, and barks of plants, which impart an array of flavors, fragrances, and health benefits.

In this ultimate guide to herbal teas, we'll journey through everything you need to know to explore and enjoy the healing magic of herbal teas. We'll cover the fascinating history of herbal tea traditions from around the world and the myriad wellness benefits different herbal ingredients provide. You'll learn herb-by-herb profiles so you can understand the powers of chamomile, peppermint, ginger, turmeric, and many more! We'll also go over proper brewing techniques to extract the most flavor and nourishment from the herbs.

Think of this book as your passport into the rituals and remedies of herbal tea. I aim to inspire you to slow down and savor a cup of nourishing brew. Herbal teas provide an opportunity to practice everyday wellness and imbibe the natural gifts of plants. Drinking a warm mug of herbal tea feeds the body, mind, and spirit in such simple and comforting ways. Not to mention, the tastes and aromas are out of this world!

Why Drink Herbal Tea?

Before we get into the nitty-gritty details, let's examine why herbal tea deserves a permanent place in your kitchen cabinets, health routines, and best self-care practices. Here are some of the many benefits that a cup of herbal tea can provide:

Relaxation: Herbal teas made from plants like chamomile, lavender, and lemon balm are natural stress relievers. Sipping these gently fragrant teas before bed is a soothing ritual. The herbs work to calm the nervous system and quiet the mind from its constant worrying. Herbal nightcaps support healthy, restful sleep.

Immune Support: Many herbs like echinacea, elderberry, and astragalus are loaded with antimicrobial and anti-inflammatory compounds. Incorporating these herbs into your diet strengthens your defenses against viruses, bacteria, and harmful inflammation. Herbal teas are an easy preventative health measure against seasonal colds and flus.

Digestive Aid: Plants such as peppermint, ginger, and licorice root gently soothe away tummy troubles. Enjoying a cup after meals can help alleviate indigestion, nausea, gas, and discomfort. The herbs provide anti-inflammatory, antibacterial, and muscle-relaxing effects.

Detoxification: Herbs like dandelion, nettle, and burdock work as natural diuretics and liver cleansers. Drinking teas made with these herbs may help flush toxins and excess water from your system. Think of them as an everyday detox boost.

Energy Lift: For a little pick-me-up sans the caffeine, look to energizing herbs like yerba mate, guayusa, and matcha green tea. They provide steady, smooth energy inspiration from plant compounds and antioxidants. Ditch the late afternoon coffee in favor of these adaptogenic lifts!

Female Health: Many women turn to herbal infusions for menstrual support, fertility aid, and balancing hormones. Raspberry leaf, red clover, and spearmint teas are gentle allies during PMS, menstrual cramps, menopause, and beyond. Plants have supported women's wellness for centuries.

Male Health: Herbal teas can also benefit prostate health and function for men. Ingredients like saw palmetto, stinging nettle root, and pygeum bark have been shown to relieve urinary symptoms and potentially improve testosterone levels.

The options are truly limitless when it comes to the wellness perks of herbal tea. One infusion can provide antioxidants, improve digestion, relax the mind, and boost immunity all in one aromatic mug. Keep reading to begin uncovering how you can harness the benefits of plants through teas.

Chapter 1

A Brief History of Herbal Tea

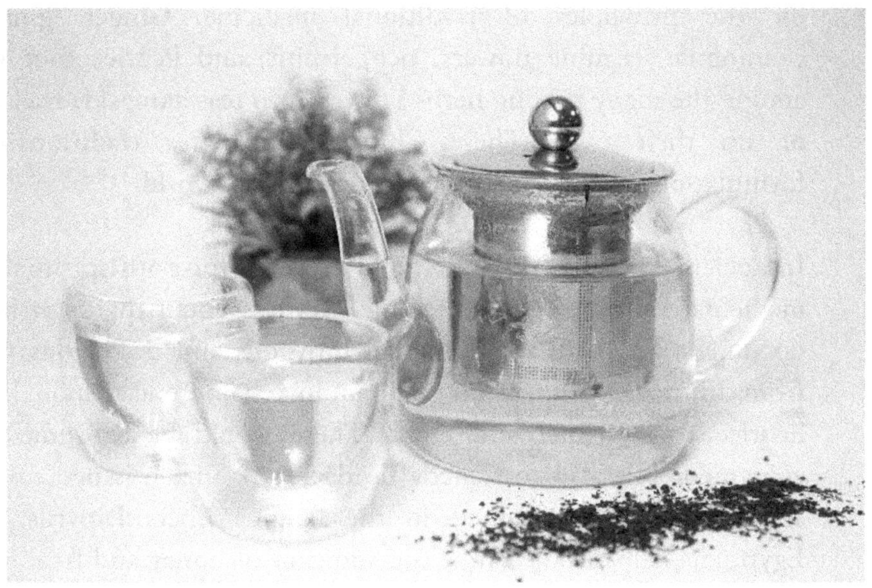

The ritual of steeping herbs, spices, roots, and other botanicals in hot water for medicinal and enjoyable consumption has an ancient history spanning back thousands of years across various cultures worldwide. From Asia to Europe, the Middle East, Africa and the Americas, humans have long recognized and utilized the healing gifts of plants, drinking them as teas for holistic well-being. Understanding this rich global history helps contextualize the traditions and benefits of herbal teas that we still enjoy today.

The first written records of herbal tea consumption date back over 5,000 years ago to ancient China, where the first Emperor Shen Nung famously discovered and promoted the drinking of tea for its medicinal properties and energizing qualities. China is considered the ancestral home of the Camellia sinensis tea plant, whose leaves and buds are used to produce true teas like green, black, white, and oolong tea. The Chinese also commonly incorporated various herbs into tea preparations to serve as remedies for specific ailments based on the principles of traditional medicine. Ginger, ginseng, chamomile, jasmine flowers, peppermint, and licorice root were among the many healing herbs brewed into teas alongside tea leaves or on their own. These Chinese herbal tea traditions and formulations would spread across Asia and the world.

In ancient Egypt, herbs were highly revered for both spiritual and medicinal purposes. Many temple carvings and papyrus writings document Egyptian use of herbal infusions and decoctions made from hibiscus, peppermint, cinnamon, chamomile, lemon balm, licorice root, fennel and more. These would be consumed for enjoyment but also to remedy headaches, stomach issues, coughs, and colds as documented in the famous Ebers Papyrus. The Egyptians helped popularize the addition of honey and fruit juices to herbal teas to balance the bitter tastes of some plants.

The practice of Ayurvedic medicine in ancient India relied heavily on herbal teas and infusions for preventing and treating disease. Traditional Ayurvedic tea preparations combined potent spices like cardamom, cloves, cinnamon, ginger, holy basil, and black peppercorn with brewed black tea and medicinal roots to create flavorsome and rejuvenating drinks. Popular masala chai tea blends reflect this ancestral knowledge. The herbs were selected and prepared based on an individual's specific health constitution and balance of doshas.

Many indigenous African tribes similarly developed a deep plant medicine tradition of harvesting abundant local herbs for infusions. Teas might contain rooibos, honeybush, hibiscus, ginger, peppercorn, flowers, and roots. They were valued for their medicinal effects and also consumed as part of community rituals and ceremonies. Knowledge of the plant's healing powers was passed down orally over generations.

In the Americas, Native American herbal tea practices evolved regionally based on local flora. Teas were derived from herbs like yaupon, bee balm, spicebush, wild thyme, pine needles, sassafras, and more. Beyond physical health, these were used in spiritual ceremonies to connect with ancestors and the earth. The Andean people in South America brewed teas from mate, guayusa, and other energizing plants native to the Amazon into tonics for vitality and mental clarity.

During the Middle Ages in Europe and Persia, monks adapted and experimented with various imported Asian herbs for their monastery gardens alongside local ingredients, developing an herbal tea tradition drawing from multiple cultures. Their formulations were passed down in ancient medicinal texts. As new herbs like lavender, chamomile, sage and mint were cultivated, they found their way into both medicinal and recreational teas. The Silk Road trade network, which connected China to Europe, spurred further exchange of herbs and tea knowledge across regions.

From ancient traditional systems of holistic health to colonial apothecaries to modern commercial blends, herbal tea history weaves a rich narrative through human civilization. While methods have evolved, the essence of carefully selecting and steeping herbs in water for therapy and enjoyment remains unchanged. As we'll explore throughout this book, herbal teas offer a delicious and accessible daily ritual that connects us to the ancient wisdom of medicinal plants.

Tea Traditions Around the World

While herbal teas trace back thousands of years in various regions globally, unique tea preparation rituals, customs, and localized ingredients have developed across cultures over time. Examining distinctive international herbal tea traditions provides insight into the plant wisdom and infusion methods used in different places that have endured into modern times. From Japanese tea ceremonies to South American mate rituals to Moroccan mint teas, diverse cultures have made tea drinking a resonant part of holistic well-being.

In China, the birthplace of tea, intricate traditions surround preparing and drinking teas for health, reflection and community. Green, black, oolong and white teas made solely from the Camellia sinensis plant take prominence, often complemented with warming Chinese herbs like jujube, ginseng, goji berry, ginger and medicinal mushrooms in complex formulations. For millennia, Chinese medicine has utilized herbal teas as preventative tonics and to treat ailments based on the unique energetics of each plant and the needs of the individual. Teahouses and tea-drinking rituals pervade Chinese culture as sites of respite, rejuvenation and connection.

The Japanese tea tradition centers around the tranquil, meditative nature of tea drinking as part of the cultural aesthetic of wabi-sabi, or finding beauty in imperfection. The intricate Japanese tea ceremony, or Chanoyu, focuses on every detail of making and presenting matcha green tea for guests as an act of hospitality, mindfulness and artistry. The preparation involves carefully choreographed steps, including the selection of garden-grown tea and ceramics, precise whisking techniques, and offering sweets to complement the bitter tea. Beyond the ceremony, green teas like sencha and gyokuro are brewed daily and appreciated for their health benefits and grounding effect.

In India, masala chai tea has become an integral part of culture, cuisine and community. This aromatic beverage combines black tea brewed with warming spices like cardamom, cinnamon, clove, ginger and black pepper, along with milk and sugar. The drink was originally used in ancient Ayurvedic medicine and then spread through South Asia by the British. Each family or street stall adds their spice blend to create a unique masala chai experience that awakens the senses and brings people together. The sweet, spicy tea is enjoyed throughout the day and offered to guests as an act of goodwill and nourishment.

The Moroccan tradition of drinking fresh spearmint tea weaves together hospitality, health and leisure. Moroccan green tea with fragrant native Nana mint is served in ornate silver teapots multiple times daily and offered to visitors as a refreshing drink that aids digestion. Tea time is a chance to take a pause, build community, and gain the medicinal benefits of mint. Across North Africa and the Middle East, drinking herb-infused green teas like peppermint, sage, and verbena grown locally is integral to culture and well-being.

Yerba mate tea is a social ritual in many South American countries, namely Argentina, Uruguay, Paraguay and Brazil, where it grows in the rainforest. Sharing mate (pronounced mah-tay) from a gourd through a metal straw with friends and family is a sign of trust, bonding, and hospitality. Originating with indigenous Guaraní tribes, yerba mate provides caffeine for sustained energy and vitality. The tea is consumed casually throughout the day, in the morning, during breaks at work, with meals, and at gatherings. Each region personalizes mate tea culture, terminology, and accouterments.

Across the African continent, herbal teas indigenous to the land infuse culture. Rooibos and honeybush tisanes enjoyed for centuries by native Khoisan tribes now constitute a national pastime for South Africans and a global export. Ethiopians partake in a unique coffee ceremony that includes burning frankincense resin and sipping spiced herbal coffee. Egyptians sip hibiscus and lemongrass teas mid-day to quench thirst and offer refreshment. These are just a sampling of distinctive herbal tea traditions connecting people to the healing, community-building and convivial aspects of plants.

From Japanese tea ceremonies to Brazilian mate circles to Moroccan hospitality, herbal tea rituals serve as time-honored traditions that provide nourishment for the body while connecting us to other cultures. Experiencing global tea practices allows us to broaden our palates and understanding of tea's place in holistic wellness.

Modern Scientific Understanding of Herbal Tea

While herbal tea traditions stretch back millennia, modern scientific research in the past decades has strived to understand better and validate the empirical knowledge passed down about medicinal herbs' mechanisms, bioactive compounds, and measurable health effects. Rigorous studies aimed at identifying the biological activities and pharmacological actions of commonly used tea herbs provide greater insight into ancient plant wisdom. Findings confirm many traditional uses while also uncovering new therapeutic properties.

For instance, clinical trials substantiate the anti-inflammatory properties of turmeric, rooibos, and green tea, verifying their traditional Ayurvedic and Chinese medicine applications for arthritis, joint pain, and autoimmune conditions. The antioxidant, antimicrobial and antiviral capacities of elderberry, echinacea, olive leaf, and astragalus to fight upper respiratory infections and flu are also evidenced through clinical research. Chamomile and lemon balm's anti-anxiety effects on the central nervous system align with centuries of employing them for relaxation and sleep.

Modern analysis can pinpoint exactly which bioactive molecules are responsible for different herbs' impacts, ranging from polyphenols, flavonoids, and catechins to terpenes, glycosides, and alkaloids. For example, experts attribute chamomile's calming nature to a flavonoid called apigenin, while caffeine and theophylline give guayusa leaves their energizing effect. Knowing the chemical profiles of herbs allows us to understand better why and how they benefit wellness.

While most herbal tea components have been traditionally viewed as safe at typical culinary doses, research illuminates potential side effects and contraindications worth noting. Interactions between herbs and pharmaceuticals may also occur, underscoring the need for awareness. For instance, licorice root can exacerbate hypertension and heart conditions. Verifying safety alongside efficacy is key.

The scientific examination also unlocks new potential wellness applications for herbs not traditionally used for health, like hibiscus' ability to lower blood pressure. Unbiased research detached from any folklore or cultural tea practices allows unique herb properties and combinations to emerge. The synergistic interaction between turmeric and black pepper to increase curcumin absorption was realized this way.

An Overview of Potential Wellness Benefits

Sipping herbal teas has long been valued as a simple ritual that provides soothing sensory pleasure along with an array of potential wellness benefits. Modern research has begun to shed light on the wide range of therapeutic properties various botanicals possess when brewed into tea. While claims should be verified, centuries of traditional use and contemporary studies suggest herbal teas may aid well-being in numerous ways. Getting acquainted with some of the key benefits can help guide your exploration into herbal teas for preventative health and gentle healing.

Relaxation: Many beloved herbs like chamomile, lavender, lemon balm, and catnip have mild sedative, tranquilizing properties that can help relax both mind and body. Their natural plant compounds interact with receptors in the brain to promote calmness. Sipping teas made with these herbs before bedtime can ease anxiety and insomnia to pave the way for a deeper sleep. During the day, they can provide a sense of focused calm to relieve stress.

Immune Support: Herbs like echinacea, elderberry, and astragalus contain antioxidants, polyphenols, and polysaccharides that can help strengthen immune function. Regularly drinking medicinal herb teas may help protect against colds, flu, and infections by supporting healthy immune responses. Adaptogens like ginseng, licorice, and holy basil in tea can also buffer the effects of stress on immunity.

Detoxification: Specific herbs support the body's natural detoxification processes through organs like the liver, kidneys, and lymphatic system. Milk thistle, dandelion, nettle, burdock, and red clover help flush toxins and provide antioxidants. Enjoying these herbal teas supports gentle cleansing from within.

Digestive Aid: The anti-inflammatory, antimicrobial, and carminative properties of herbs like peppermint, ginger, fennel, licorice, and chamomile can help ease digestive issues when brewed into tea. They relax gut spasms, reduce gas, and alleviate nausea, heartburn, stomach pain, and bloating for more comfortable digestion.

Women's Health: Teas made with herbs like red raspberry leaf, red clover, evening primrose, and Dong Quai have been traditionally used to support women's reproductive health and hormonal balance. They are thought to help ease PMS, menopause symptoms, and fertility issues and provide comfort during menstruation.

Circulatory Aid: Herbs like hawthorn berries, ginger, and garlic can support healthy blood flow and circulation when consumed as tea. They may also help manage blood pressure levels and cholesterol markers. Enjoying these teas regularly promotes cardiovascular wellness.

Antioxidant Protection: Abundant antioxidants from herbs like green tea, rosehip, lemongrass, and hibiscus neutralize free radicals that can damage cells. This helps prevent accelerated aging, inflammation, and disease. Brewing high-antioxidant herbs into teas makes it easy to reap protective benefits.

Energy Promotion: Herbs like guayusa, yerba mate, ginseng, and matcha green tea contain caffeine and adaptogenic compounds that promote sustained energy, alertness, and vitality when consumed as teas. They provide an alternative to coffee for a morning or afternoon pick-me-up.

Joint Support: Anti-inflammatory herbs like turmeric, green tea, nettle leaf, and pine bark can help ease joint pain and arthritis when taken regularly. Nutritive ingredients also support bone health. Enjoying these herbal allies may bring comfort to aging joints.

The range of wellness benefits different medicinal herbs can provide is truly remarkable. Drinking tea daily offers a delicious preventative health boost alongside targeted relief as needed. Listen to your body and notice how different herbal teas make you feel. Their gentle support can optimize wellbeing.

Sourcing High-Quality Ingredients

When brewing herbal teas, source the highest quality ingredients you can find for the greatest health benefits and most delicious flavors. Seek out reputable suppliers that ethically harvest herbs, use chemical-free growing practices, and process leaves, roots, and flowers minimally after harvest. With herbal teas, quality is key. Follow these tips for finding top-tier teas:

Focus on organic. Organic farming prohibits synthetic pesticides and fertilizers that can concentrate in herbs and pass on in brewed tea. While more costly, organic herbs are ideal to avoid ingesting any residues or toxins. Even just selecting organic for herbs you consume frequently can make a difference.

Know your grower. Research companies producing herbal tea products to learn about their ethics and processes. Many superior tea suppliers post extensive details about their sustainable farms and harvest practices. Connecting to a tea's origins builds trust.

Buy loose leaves. Whole, loose-leaf herbal teas typically offer far better quality and flavor than pre-bagged options. You can inspect, smell, and admire the whole leaves. Loose teas also give more control over blend ratios.

Read the ingredients. For any pre-made tea blends, read the label closely to make sure no strange additives, flavorings or unnecessary ingredients are included. Watch for natural versus artificial flavors.

Check expiration dates. Herbal tea leaves and flowers can lose aromatic essential oils and potency over time. Avoid old products by checking expiration or best-by dates on packaging. Shop at markets with good ingredient turnover.

Inspect appearance. Quality dried herbs should retain much of their original color, aroma, shape, and texture. Avoid dull, broken herbs with faded color or hardly any scent, which indicates age.

Smell the aroma. Take a good whiff of dried herbs, and they should smell vibrant, not musty. Rich, grassy, floral and earthy aromas signal healthier herbs. Trust your nose.

Taste the flavor. High-quality herbs and flowers should taste robust, not weak. Aim for bright, complex flavors rather than dull or flat-tasting tea. The difference is striking.

Consider fair trade. Seek out fair trade certified herbal teas whenever possible to support sustainable livelihoods for small-scale farmers worldwide.

Shop local. Visiting a local herbal apothecary allows you to discover small-batch blended teas and learn about the sourcing process firsthand.

With an abundance of herbal teas now available, put some care into finding ones that resonate. Support companies dedicated to purity, quality, and sustainable practices. Your cup will brim with more flavor and balanced nourishment.

Proper Storage for Maximum Freshness

To retain the highest quality and effectiveness of your herbal tea ingredients, proper storage is key. When stored incorrectly, delicate leaves, flowers, roots, and seeds can lose flavor, aroma and beneficial compounds over time. By keeping herbs in optimal conditions, you preserve their precious essences and maximize shelf life. Follow these best practices for locking in freshness:

Guard against air, light, and moisture. The triple enemies of fresh herbs are air oxidation, light exposure, and ambient moisture. Keep teas in opaque, airtight containers away from direct light and humidity. Opaque glass jars work great.

Mind the temperature. Store teas in a cool, dry spot away from heat sources like ovens, stoves, and heating vents. The ideal range is 50°F to 70°F. Avoid temperature fluctuations.

Separate and label. If combining multiple loose-leaf teas in one container, use divider inserts to separate them and prevent blending. Label jars for easy identification.

Practice first-in, first-out. Adopt first-in, first-out organization by placing newly purchased teas behind older ones. Pull from the front and use the oldest first for best quality.

Check for freshness. Periodically smell and visually inspect stored teas for fading aroma, color changes, or moisture clumping. Refresh stale inventory to maintain flavor.

Keep herbs whole. Leave herbs whole rather than grinding them into powders, which degrades compounds. Breaking leaves just before steeping releases oils.

Don't refrigerate most herbs. While refrigeration extends life for some ingredients like roots, it ruins leaves. The condensation introduced causes deterioration.
Freeze delicate herbs. To extend the lifespan of more fragile herbs like hibiscus, rosehips, and basil, consider freezing. Use ice cube trays.

Transfer to smaller vessels. Once opened, transfer bulk teas to smaller containers with less air space. Oxygen accelerates staling.

Buy smaller quantities. For herbs you use infrequently, but just enough to last several months to avoid waste from expiry.

Know expiration dates. Even properly stored herbs lose potency over 1-2 years. Reference expiration or Best By dates and renew the stock.

By becoming a steward of your herbal collection and drinking teas promptly, you reap the optimal vitality from each precious leaf. Proper storage rewards you with endless cups of nourishment.

Chapter 2
Herbal Teas for Energy, Focus and Vitality

Feeling mentally sharp, focused and energized throughout your day is crucial for peak performance. Many people rely on coffee for stimulating effects, but over time, caffeine can cause jitteriness and exhaustion. Certain herbal teas offer a natural source of sustainable energy, mental clarity, and productivity-enhancing benefits without the unwanted side effects of too much coffee.

Plants like guarana, yerba mate, green tea, and guayusa contain caffeine-like compounds that provide a smooth energy boost without jitters or crashes. Herbs like peppermint, lemon balm and rosemary increase alertness. Adaptogens like gynostemma and maca help combat fatigue and stress. Discover how incorporating these top herbal brews into your routine can elevate your vitality, productivity, motivation and mental performance all day long.

Invigorating Mint and Lemon Verbena Tea

This refreshing caffeine-free tea combo is perfect for boosting energy and focus any time of the day without disrupting sleep cycles. Peppermint contains menthol, which stimulates receptors in the brain associated with increased mental clarity. Lemon verbena elevates mood and concentration while also easing tension.

To make a cup, simply add 2 tablespoons of dried peppermint leaves and 1 tablespoon of dried lemon verbena leaves to a tea ball. Steep in 8 oz hot water for 5-7 minutes. The bright, uplifting aroma will awaken your mind as the herbs gently stimulate circulation and breathing. Mint and lemon verbena make a tasty pick-me-up beverage without the caffeine crash later.

Green Tea and Lemon Balm Elixir for Gentle Focus

For those sensitive to caffeine, this meadow-like infusion provides sustained concentration and calm productivity. Green tea has just enough caffeine to enhance mental acuity without being overstimulating. Lemon balm helps maintain focus by relaxing the mind and easing anxiety.

Gently simmer 1 tablespoon of dried green tea leaves and 2 tablespoons of dried lemon balm leaves in 8 oz water for 7 minutes. Avoid overheating green tea as extreme temperatures diminish the catechins. The delicate flavor and soothing aroma promote relaxation, while the low dose of caffeine provides just enough mental and physical stamina to power through your day.

Yerba Mate, Cacao and Maca Energy Tonic

Yerba mate delivers the energizing benefits of coffee minus the jitteriness, thanks to its unique blend of xanthine alkaloids. Cacao contains mild stimulants for further brain boosting. Maca balances the effects with adaptogenic, hormone-regulating properties.

Stir together 2 tablespoons yerba mate, 1 tablespoon cacao powder, 1 teaspoon maca powder. Steep in 8 oz hot (not boiling) water for 5-7 minutes. The earthy combination provides sustained energy, mood lift, and mental drive. Yerba mate also enhances focus, learning, and memory. Drink this tea latte as a coffee substitute that doesn't sacrifice energy.

Classic Black Tea Chai with Cardamom

This aromatic, gently caffeinated tea is a staple in Ayurvedic medicine for its energizing warmth and digestive benefits. Black tea contains just enough caffeine to enhance alertness without overstimulation. Cardamom boosts circulation and blood flow to the brain for improved concentration and motivation.

Simmer 2 black tea bags, 6 green cardamom pods, 4 cloves and 1 cinnamon stick in 2 cups milk or nondairy milk for 5 minutes. Remove from heat and add 1/4 teaspoon vanilla. The spicy-sweet chai latte provides a steady energy supply for several hours, making it great for sipping at your desk to stay productive.

Ginger and Turmeric Golden Latte for Immune Energy
Soothing and anti-inflammatory, this vibrant elixir leverages the stimulant properties of ginger together with the adaptogenic benefits of turmeric for sustained energy and immunity. Ginger energizes the body and mind while easing aches, boosting circulation and improving digestion. Turmeric provides an anti-stress antidepressant lift.

Heat 2 cups of non dairy milk just below a boil. Whisk in 1 teaspoon of turmeric, 1 tablespoon of grated ginger, 1 tablespoon of maple syrup and a dash of black pepper. The earthy, savory golden latte delivers a steady energy supply that counters stress and bolsters the immune response, making it ideal for avoiding burnout during busy times.

Guayusa Tea Sweetened with Maple Syrup

This next-level energy tea is made from the guayusa holly leaf, which is packed with caffeine, theanine, and chlorogenic acid for smooth, sustained energy and mental stamina. Guayusa provides the alertness of coffee without jitteriness or an evening energy crash. Its pleasant, mellow flavor benefits from a touch of natural sweetness.

Steep 2 tablespoons of loose guayusa leaves in 8 oz hot (not boiling) water for 4-5 minutes. Strain the leaves, then stir in 1 tablespoon pure maple syrup. The maple perfectly balances guayusa's complex flavor. Just 1-2 mugs provide hours of sustained mental clarity and physical energy minus the buzz and crash of excessive caffeine.

Beauty Berry and Hibiscus Antioxidant Blend
Give your energy levels an antioxidant supercharge with this fruity, floral infusion. Beauty berries contain antioxidants called anthocyanins that strengthen immunity, fight inflammation and neutralize harmful free radicals caused by stress. Hibiscus boosts energy by lowering blood pressure and providing hydration.

Simmer 4-5 dried beauty berries and 2 tablespoons of hibiscus petals in 8 oz water for 7-10 minutes. Steep green tea leaves in the brew if a touch of caffeine is desired. Sweeten with honey or maple syrup. Sip this vibrant infusion during stressful times as an energizing pick-me-up full of protective antioxidants.

Discover more get-up-and-go by exploring the wide world of energizing herbs and botanicals. Move beyond coffee and experience sustained energy, stamina and mental clarity from naturally caffeinated teas and superfood elixirs. With the right energizing brews by your side, you'll stay focused and motivated to take on whatever comes your way.

More Naturally Caffeinated Teas for Sustained Energy

Maintaining energy, productivity and motivation throughout busy work days can be challenging without relying on excessive caffeine. Fortunately, nature provides many herbs and plants containing compounds that deliver smooth, jitter-free stimulation for sustained mental and physical stamina.

Beyond traditional teas, there are many refreshing botanicals to explore that provide a natural energy boost, including yerba mate, guayusa, guarana and kratom leaf. Adaptogens like astragalus, ashwagandha, and cacao also counter fatigue. And nootropics such as ginkgo, gotu kola and bacopa enhance cognitive function. Discover more ways to boost your daily drive with these energizing, focus-enhancing herbal brews.

Cacao, Maca and Mesquite Energy Latte
This creamy caffeinated drink leverages the stimulant properties of raw cacao together with maca for sustained energy and stamina. Cacao contains theobromine, which provides gentle stimulation of the central nervous system. Maca boosts mood and endurance. Mesquite balances the sweetness.

Heat 2 cups of non dairy milk over medium just until steaming. Whisk in 2 tablespoons raw cacao powder, 1 tablespoon maca powder and 1 tablespoon mesquite powder. The delicious mood-enhancing latte provides mental and physical energy along with an antidepressant lift to get you through the daily grind.

Guarana and Ginseng Berry Boost:
This tropical pick-me-up harnesses the caffeine-like effects of guarana paired with the adaptogenic energy of ginseng. Guarana seeds contain guarana, which stimulates the brain much like caffeine

but with fewer jitters. Ginseng further enhances physical stamina and mental performance.

Steep 2 tablespoons of guarana seed powder and 1 tablespoon of dried ginseng berry powder in 8 oz hot water for 5 minutes. Sweeten with a bit of honey if desired. The berry-flavored beverage provides smooth stimulation with no crash later. Guarana's slower-releasing caffeine also prolongs the energizing effects.

Yerba Mate Citrus Spritzer
This lightly sweet iced tea showcases yerba mate's energizing properties in a refreshing beverage. Yerba mate delivers caffeine along with theanine for sustained energy, mental clarity, and productivity. Tangy citrus oils balance the earthy, herbaceous flavor.

Brew 2 tablespoons yerba mate tea in 8 oz hot water for 5 minutes. Steep 1 orange wedge, 1 lemon wedge, and several mint leaves. Cool, then strain over ice and stir in 2 tablespoons of fresh orange juice. For just 36 calories a glass, this brisk iced tea offers caffeine-freebies as a satisfying mimosa-hour substitute.

Turmeric and Ginger Immunity Booster
Spicy, fragrant, and ultra-soothing, this vibrant elixir leverages anti-inflammatory turmeric and ginger to combat fatigue and bolster immune defenses. Turmeric provides an antidepressant antianxiety lift while ginger stimulates blood flow and energy. The combination wards off stress and prevents burnout.

Gently simmer ½ teaspoon turmeric powder and 1 tablespoon grated fresh ginger in 16 oz nondairy milk for 5-7 minutes. Strain if desired and add a dash of cinnamon and black pepper. The soothing brew energizes and grounds the mind, making it the perfect daily drink for self-care and immune support.

Gotu Kola and Bacopa Brain Booster
This earthy infusion optimizes cognitive function using two time-honored Ayurvedic herbs. Gotu kola enhances memory, learning, and concentration. Bacopa improves information retention and mental endurance. The perfect tea for staying mentally sharp.

Place 1 tablespoon gotu kola, 1 tablespoon bacopa, 1 teaspoon fennel seeds, and 1 crushed cardamom pod in a tea infuser. Steep in 6-8 oz hot water for 5 minutes. Sweeten with honey if desired. Sip this brew daily for enhanced neuroplasticity, productivity, motivation, and work performance.

Holy Basil and Lemon Balm Stress Reliever
Holy basil and lemon balm make a soothing, adaptogenic tea that helps counter the effects of chronic stress for renewed energy and stamina. Holy basil contains compounds that regulate cortisol levels. Lemon balm calms anxiety and tension.

Steep 2 tablespoons each of dried holy basil leaves and lemon balm leaves in 8 oz boiling water for 7 minutes. Adding some raw honey brings out the herbs' lemony-sweet essence while further easing stress. Drink a cup or two daily during stressful times to give your energy levels and resilience a boost.

Rosemary Mint No-Doz Beverage
This aromatic infusion leverages natural stimulants in rosemary and the acute alertness boost of mint. Carnosic acid in rosemary improves cognitive function. Mint's menthol jolts your mind awake. An excellent afternoon pick-me-up beverage without any crashes.

Steep 2-3 fresh rosemary sprigs and 5-6 fresh mint leaves (or 1 tablespoon dried mint) in 8 oz boiling water for 5-7 minutes. Sweeten with a spoonful of honey if desired. The refreshing brew stimulates circulation while enhancing mental clarity, memory, and concentration for effortless afternoon productivity.

Kratom and Black Tea Energy Blend
Native to Thailand and Malaysia, the kratom leaf contains compounds that provide a caffeine-like stimulant effect for sustained energy. Its mild alkaloids offer a smooth lift without jitters. Black tea's low caffeine provides further gentle stimulation.

Combine 2 teaspoons of ground kratom leaf and 1 black tea bag in an infuser. Steep in 6-8 oz boiling water for 10 minutes. Remove the tea bag after 2 minutes if a milder caffeine dose is preferred. Kratom's stimulating compounds pair perfectly with black tea for productivity.

The possibilities are endless when leveraging energizing botanicals in clever beverage recipes. Look beyond coffee and explore the wide world of plant-based options for stimulating elixirs. With sustained energy from herbs, adaptogens, teas, and superfoods, you'll stay motivated and focused every minute of your day.

Boosting Energy and Productivity with Herbal Infusions

Maintaining high energy, focus, and motivation levels can be challenging during busy work days without relying on excessive caffeine. Luckily, certain herbs and botanicals contain compounds that provide smooth, sustained stimulation for increased productivity, mental clarity, and physical stamina.

Beyond just caffeinated teas, nature offers many invigorating plants and superfoods for making energizing beverages without the crash later. Adaptogens like Rhodiola and ashwagandha fight fatigue. Herbs like spearmint and rosemary provide acute concentration. And nootropics such as gotu kola and ginkgo biloba optimize cognitive function. Discover more ways to upgrade your daily drive with these enlightening brews.

Yerba Mate and Mint Refreshment Beverage
This lively infusion pairs yerba mate's gentle caffeine lift with the refreshing notes of mint and citrus. Yerba mate contains xanthines that stimulate focus and mental clarity. Mint's aromatic oils awaken the mind. Together they provide hours of crisp, sustained energy.

Steep 2 tablespoons of loose yerba mate and 5-6 crushed mint leaves in 6-8 oz hot water (not boiling) for 5 minutes. Add the juice of 1/2 lemon or lime wedge. Sweeten with honey or stevia to taste. The bright tea offers a revitalizing caffeine-free pick-me-up any time of day.

Matcha Green Tea Energy Latte
This velvety latte harnesses the stimulating properties of matcha's natural caffeine, L-theanine, and epigallocatechin gallate (EGCG) for sustained energy and mental stamina. Matcha provides caffeine's cognitive boost without anxiety or crashes. Non-dairy milk adds creaminess.

Whisk 1 teaspoon matcha powder into 2 oz hot water until frothy. Heat 8 oz non-dairy milk until steaming and pour into the matcha paste, whisking again until frothy. The antioxidant-rich latte promotes relaxation, focus, memory, and metabolism. An excellent coffee substitute.

Moringa and Peppermint Productivity Enhancer
This refreshing infusion combines the mild stimulant properties of moringa with alertness-enhancing mint. Moringa contains caffeine along with tyrosine and amino acids to increase energy naturally. Peppermint's menthol jolts the mind awake.

Steep 1 tablespoon dried moringa leaf powder and 2 tablespoons fresh peppermint leaves in 6-8 oz boiling water for 5-7 minutes. Sweeten with honey if desired. The bright flavors stimulate senses and enhance blood flow. Drink daily for productivity sans the coffee jitters.

Ginseng, Garcinia and Cinnamon Metabolism Tea
This warming tea blend leverages ginger, garcinia cambogia and cinnamon for increased energy expenditure and fat burning. Ginseng boosts metabolism and energy levels. Garcinia contains HCA which helps suppress appetite. Cinnamon regulates blood glucose.

Simmer 1 teaspoon dried ginseng root, 1 teaspoon garcinia powder and 1 cinnamon stick in 2 cups of water for 15 minutes. Strain and add lemon if desired. Drink warm or chilled. The spiced tea helps increase fat burning, especially when drunk 30 minutes before exercise for amplified results.

Holy Basil and Rhodiola Antioxidant Chai
This spiced elixir combines adaptogenic herbs and black tea for a sustained energy supply and stress support. Holy basil and rhodiola combat fatigue while black tea gently stimulates. Cardamom and cinnamon provide circulation and blood flow benefits.

Herbal Allies for Increased Energy and Productivity

Having sufficient mental clarity, motivation and stamina to tackle each day's demands and achieve goals can be challenging without relying on excessive stimulants. However, nature provides many botanical options for crafting beverages that deliver jitter-free, sustained energy, without the dreaded caffeine crash.

Beyond just caffeinated teas, adaptogens like eleuthero and ashwagandha counter stress-induced fatigue. Concentration-sharpening nootropics such as ginkgo, bacopa, and gotu kola enhance cognitive function. And invigorating herbs like guayusa, yerba mate and kratom provide smooth stimulation. Discover more ways to upgrade your daily drive with these enlightening infusions.

No-Doz Thai Iced Green Tea

This lightly sweet Thai-style green tea provides a gentle yet lasting caffeine lift thanks to natural phytochemicals like L-theanine. Brimming with antioxidants, it delivers sustained energy and mental stamina without jitters or anxiety. A fantastic afternoon productivity booster.

Steep 2 green tea bags and 2 lemongrass stalks in 4 cups boiling water for 5 minutes. Remove herbs and chill the tea. Sweeten with 2 tablespoons of honey and pour over ice. Add fresh ginger root slices and mint leaves. The Thai flavors perfectly balanced green tea's mellow caffeine kick.

Yerba Mate and Lime Refresh-Mint

Yerba Mate never disappoints when you need to refuel your energy levels. Its unique mix of xanthines like caffeine and theophylline provides hours of clean mental focus. Mint and lime add an extra sensory awakening. A great coffee alternative any time of day.

Steep 2 tablespoons of loose yerba mate and a handful of crushed mint leaves in 6-8 oz hot water for 5 minutes. Strain then add the juice of 1 lime wedge for a bright, uplifting citrus twist. The mate delivers sustained energy while the mint-lime combo awakens the mind.

Turmeric, Maca, and Mesquite Elixir
This earthy elixir leverages the adaptogenic energy-boosting trio of turmeric, maca, and mesquite. Turmeric provides an uplifting antidepressant lift to combat stress and fatigue. Maca balances hormones for sustained stamina. Mesquite balances the sweetness.

Whisk 1 teaspoon turmeric, 1 tablespoon maca powder, and 2 teaspoons mesquite powder into 2 cups of warm non dairy milk. The aromatic spices deliver sustained energy, mood enhancement, and medicinal benefits. An excellent afternoon drink for a productivity pick-me-up without caffeine.

Iced Hibiscus, Orange, and Rosemary Alertness Tisane

This vibrant infusion provides a gentle cognitive boost using antioxidants, aromatics, and adaptogens. Vitamin C-rich hibiscus and orange energize immunity. Rosemary's carnosic acid improves concentration and memory. A refreshing iced tea for summer productivity.

Brew 2 hibiscus tea bags, 1 orange slice, and 1 rosemary sprig in 4 cups of just-boiled water for 7 minutes. Remove herbs, chill, and then add 2 tablespoons of orange juice. Sweeten with honey and pour over ice. Sip the bright rosemary-citrus tea as an afternoon refreshment to turn brain fog into clarity.

Ashwagandha and Holy Basil Adaptogenic Chai

This aromatic twist on chai combats stress-induced exhaustion using adaptogens ashwagandha and holy basil. Black tea provides just enough caffeine for sustained energy. Traditional Ayurvedic spices boost circulation. The perfect fuel for pushing through daily demands.

Simmer 2 black tea bags, 1 cinnamon stick, 1 teaspoon ashwagandha powder, 1 teaspoon holy basil and 6 green cardamom pods in 16 oz nondairy milk for 5 minutes. Strain and sweeten with honey to taste. Sip the brew hot to promote calm productivity all day long.

Iced Pineapple Mint Energizing Oasis
This sunny infusion blends naturally sweet pineapple and awakening mint into a revitalizing iced tea loaded with vitamin C. Pineapple energizes immunity while providing antioxidants to combat inflammation and stress. Mint's aromatic oils stimulate alertness.

Steep 4-5 pineapple mint tea bags in 4 cups boiling water for 5-7 minutes. Remove tea bags, chill overnight, and add 2 cups of pineapple juice in the morning. Sweeten to taste with honey and pour over ice for an uplifting caffeine-free fuel.

Cacao, Reishi, and Maca Elixir
Raw cacao and reishi contain compounds that provide a natural energy and mood lift. Cacao is rich in methylxanthines like theobromine. Reishi offers adaptogenic antioxidants. Maca balances the bittersweet flavors while boosting stamina.

Whisk together 2 tablespoons of raw cacao powder, 1 tablespoon of reishi extract powder, and 1 tablespoon of maca powder. Heat in 16 oz non dairy milk, without boiling, until frothy. Sweeten to taste.

The delicious elixir provides steady energy, mental clarity, and resilience for tackling daily tasks.

Lemongrass Kratom Energy Spritzer
This refreshingly tart drink harnesses the stimulated effects of kratom's alkaloids together with circulation-boosting lemongrass. Kratom provides a smooth lift similar to caffeine. Lemongrass enhances blood flow and oxygenation. A fantastic afternoon pick-me-up.

Steep 2 teaspoons crushed kratom leaf and 1 sliced lemongrass stalk in 6-8 oz hot water for 10 minutes. Strain then add fresh lemon juice for tangy citrus notes to balance the earthy flavors. Serve chilled over ice for an uplifting boost minus the crash later.

The possibilities are endless when utilizing nature's bounty of botanicals, herbs, and superfoods for crafting energizing beverages that awaken body and mind. Look beyond just coffee and caffeinated tea to elevate your productivity, creativity, and daily performance in healthy ways. The energizing infusion options are limited only by your imagination!

Herbal Allies for Increased Energy and Productivity

Having sufficient mental clarity, motivation, and stamina to tackle each day's demands and achieve goals can be challenging without relying on excessive stimulants. However, nature provides many botanical options for crafting beverages that deliver jitter-free, sustained energy, without the dreaded caffeine crash.

Beyond just caffeinated teas, adaptogens like eleuthero and ashwagandha counter stress-induced fatigue. Concentration-sharpening nootropics such as ginkgo, bacopa, and gotu kola enhance cognitive function. And invigorating herbs like guayusa, yerba mate, and kratom provide smooth stimulation. Discover more ways to upgrade your daily drive with these enlightening infusions.

No-Doz Thai Iced Green Tea

This lightly sweet Thai-style green tea provides a gentle yet lasting caffeine lift thanks to natural phytochemicals like L-theanine. Brimming with antioxidants, it delivers sustained energy and mental stamina without jitters or anxiety. A fantastic afternoon productivity booster. To make this refreshing pick-me-up, steep 2 green tea bags and 2 lemongrass stalks in 4 cups of boiling water for 5 minutes. Remove the herbs and chill the tea. Sweeten with 2 tablespoons of honey and pour over ice. Add fresh ginger root slices and mint leaves for authentic Thai flavor. The zesty citrus and ginger flavors perfectly balance green tea's mellow caffeine kick.

Yerba Mate and Lime Refresh-Mint

Yerba mate never disappoints when you need to refuel your energy levels. Its unique mix of xanthines like caffeine and theophylline provide hours of clean mental focus. Mint and lime add an extra sensory wakening. A great coffee alternative any time of day. To make this stimulating infusion, steep 2 tablespoons of loose yerba mate and a handful of crushed mint leaves in 6-8 oz hot water for 5 minutes. Strain then add the juice of 1 lime wedge for a bright, uplifting citrus twist. The mate delivers sustained energy while the mint-lime combo awakens the mind.

Turmeric, Maca and Mesquite Elixir

This earthy elixir leverages the adaptogenic energy-boosting trio of turmeric, maca and mesquite. Turmeric provides an uplifting antidepressant lift to combat stress and fatigue. Maca balances hormones for sustained stamina. Mesquite balances the sweetness.

Simply whisk 1 teaspoon turmeric, 1 tablespoon maca powder and 2 teaspoons mesquite powder into 2 cups of warm non dairy milk. The aromatic spices deliver sustained energy, mood enhancement and medicinal benefits. An excellent afternoon drink for a productivity pick-me-up without caffeine.

This vibrant infusion provides a gentle cognitive boost using antioxidants, aromatics and adaptogens. Vitamin C-rich hibiscus and orange energize immunity. Rosemary's carnosic acid improves concentration and memory. A refreshing iced tea for summer productivity. To make this sensory-awakening infusion, brew 2 hibiscus tea bags, 1 orange slice, and 1 rosemary sprig in 4 cups of just-boiled water for 7 minutes. Remove the herbs, chill, and then add 2 tablespoons of orange juice. Sweeten with honey and pour over ice. Sip the bright rosemary-citrus tea as an afternoon refreshment to turn brain fog into clarity.

Ashwagandha and Holy Basil Adaptogenic Chai
This aromatic twist on chai combats stress-induced exhaustion using adaptogens ashwagandha and holy basil. Black tea provides just enough caffeine for sustained energy. Traditional Ayurvedic spices boost circulation. The perfect fuel for pushing through daily demands. For this energizing masala chai, simmer 2 black tea bags, 1 cinnamon stick, 1 teaspoon ashwagandha powder, 1 teaspoon holy basil, and 6 green cardamom pods in 16 oz nondairy milk for 5 minutes. Strain and sweeten with honey to taste. Sip the brew hot to promote calm productivity all day long.

Iced Pineapple Mint Energizing Oasis
This sunny infusion blends naturally sweet pineapple and awakening mint into a revitalizing iced tea loaded with vitamin C. Pineapple energizes immunity while providing antioxidants to combat inflammation and stress. Mint's aromatic oils stimulate

alertness. To make this tropical drink, steep 4-5 pineapple mint tea bags in 4 cups boiling water for 5-7 minutes. Remove tea bags, chill overnight, and add 2 cups of pineapple juice in the morning. Sweeten to taste with honey and pour over ice for an uplifting caffeine-free fuel.

Cacao, Reishi, and Maca Elixir
Raw cacao and reishi contain compounds that provide a natural energy and mood lift. Cacao is rich in methylxanthines like theobromine. Reishi offers adaptogenic antioxidants. Maca balances the bittersweet flavors while boosting stamina. Simply whisk together 2 tablespoons of raw cacao powder, 1 tablespoon of reishi extract powder, and 1 tablespoon of maca powder. Heat in 16 oz non dairy milk, without boiling, until frothy. Sweeten to taste. The delicious elixir provides steady energy, mental clarity, and resilience for tackling daily tasks.

Lemongrass Kratom Energy Spritzer
This refreshingly tart drink harnesses the stimulated effects of kratom's alkaloids together with circulation-boosting lemongrass. Kratom provides a smooth lift similar to caffeine. Lemongrass enhances blood flow and oxygenation. A fantastic afternoon pick-me-up. To make this zesty-infused spritzer, steep 2 teaspoons of crushed kratom leaf and 1 sliced lemongrass stalk in 6-8 oz hot water for 10 minutes. Strain then add fresh lemon juice for tangy citrus notes to balance the earthy flavors. Serve chilled over ice for an uplifting boost minus the crash later.

The possibilities are endless when utilizing nature's bounty of botanicals, herbs, and superfoods for crafting energizing beverages that awaken the body and mind. Look beyond just coffee and caffeinated tea to elevate your productivity, creativity, and daily performance in healthy ways. The energizing infusion options are limited only by your imagination!

Natural Botanical Beverages for Energy, Focus, and Clarity

Achieving optimal energy levels, mental sharpness, and motivation throughout busy days without excessive stimulants can be a challenge. However, nature provides many invigorating herbs and plants for making beverages that deliver smooth, sustained energy and concentration without the dreaded caffeine crash.

Beyond traditional teas, there are many natural energizers to explore including yerba mate, kratom, moringa, and cacao. Brain-boosting nootropics such as ginkgo biloba, bacopa, and rhodiola enhance cognitive function. And adaptogens like maca, ashwagandha, and ginseng counter stress-induced fatigue. Discover more ways to upgrade your daily drive with these enlightening brews.

Minty Matcha Green Tea Latte

Give your energy levels a sustained boost from the natural phytochemicals in green tea like epigallocatechin gallate (EGCG) and L-theanine. Matcha also enhances fat burning. Frothed non-dairy milk provides a deliciously creamy texture and protein. To make this latte, whisk 1 teaspoon of matcha powder into 2 oz hot water until frothy. Heat and froth 8 oz non dairy milk, then combine it with the matcha paste. Enjoy this antioxidant-rich latte hot or chilled.

Yerba Mate Mango Pick-Me-Up

Yerba Mate never disappoints when you need an afternoon pick-me-up without the post-caffeine energy crash. Its unique mix of xanthines provides hours of sustained energy and mental stamina. Mango adds tropical sweetness along with immune-boosting vitamin C and filling fiber to balance the earthy tea. Blend 2 tablespoons yerba mate, 1 cup mango, and 1 cup water. Enjoy chilled.

Ashwagandha Rhodiola Chai Latte
This steamy chai latte leverages adaptogens ashwagandha and rhodiola to combat exhaustion while black tea provides just enough caffeine for sustained energy. Cardamom and cinnamon lend their spicy-sweet flavors to an aromatic sensory experience. Simmer 2 black tea bags with 1/2 teaspoon each of ashwagandha and rhodiola powder, 1 cinnamon stick, and 2 crushed cardamom pods in 16 oz nondairy milk for 5 minutes. Sweeten to taste and sip mindfully.

Iced Grapefruit Green Tea Metabolism Booster
This tangy citrus iced tea utilizes the powerhouse combo of green tea and grapefruit to boost fat burning. Green tea contains EGCG, which ramps up metabolism. Grapefruit provides naringenin, which reduces insulin resistance. Brew 2 green tea bags and 1 grapefruit wedge in 4 cups of water for 5 minutes, chill overnight then remove tea bags and grapefruit. Add 2 tablespoons of grapefruit juice. Enjoy this brew before your workout for amplified calorie burn.

Kratom, Cinnamon, and Almond Milk Nog
Kratom's alkaloids offer a sustained stimulation similar to caffeine to help power through busy afternoons minus the crash later. Cinnamon stabilizes blood sugar for steady energy. Nutty almond milk provides vitamin E, an essential antioxidant for combating stress. Blend 2 teaspoons of kratom powder, 1/2 teaspoon cinnamon, and 1 cup of almond milk. Heat gently and enjoy the warmth.

Passionfruit Guayusa Antioxidant Cooler
Refresh and re-energize with this fruity iced tea featuring antioxidant-rich guayusa holly leaf for sustained energy. Guayusa

provides caffeine along with theanine for mental clarity. Passionfruit boosts vitamin C intake while providing neurotransmitter-enhancing choline. Steep 2 tablespoons of loose guayusa leaves in 4 cups of boiling water for 5 minutes. Allow to cool, then add 1/4 cup passionfruit juice and sweeten to taste. Enjoy this tropical cooler over ice.

Chai Masala Latte with Reishi Mushroom
This steamy, spiced chai latte features energizing reishi mushrooms instead of coffee for a warming pick-me-up any time of day. Reishi contains triterpenoids that provide anti-fatigue benefits to combat stress and improve cognitive function. Traditional chai spices like cardamom, cinnamon, and clove boost circulation while black tea offers gentle stimulation. Simmer 2 chai tea bags with 1 tablespoon reishi powder, a dash of cloves, 1 cinnamon stick, and 2 bruised cardamom pods in 16 oz nondairy milk for 5 minutes. Sweeten to taste.

The possibilities are endless when leveraging energizing herbs, teas, spices, and superfoods. Look beyond coffee to craft botanical-based beverages that awaken, motivate, and bring sustained clarity throughout busy days. With the right natural stimulants and brain-boosting adaptogens in your cup, you'll stay focused and productive all day long.

47

Chapter 3

Tension Tamer - Chamomile and Lavender

As we go through our daily lives, it's easy to get wound up tight with stress, anxiety, and tension. Our fast-paced modern world is full of traffic jams, work deadlines, family obligations, and information overload from smartphones and social media. This non-stop stimulation can make us feel frantic, overwhelmed, and ready to snap. Of course, no one wants to live like that!

When we're tied up in knots, our health and happiness suffer. Tension contributes to headaches, muscle pain, insomnia, irritability, fatigue, and more. To break free, we need to actively calm and soothe our nervous system. One of the most pleasant ways to relax and unwind is by sipping on a hot cup of herbal tea. The warmth, aroma, and ritual of preparing tea are inherently calming. Even better, many herbs have natural sedative and anxiety-relieving properties that promote deep relaxation.

One of the most renowned tension-taming teas is a blend of chamomile and lavender. These two herbs have been used for centuries to ease anxiety and lull people into tranquil slumber. Gentle chamomile has long been nicknamed "nature's Valium" for its mild sedative qualities. Lavender lends its sweet floral perfume along with potent anti-anxiety and mood-lifting benefits. Together, they make a powerfully soothing brew.

Chamomile is made from the dried flowers of Matricaria chamomilla, a member of the Asteraceae plant family. Often brewed alone as a tea, it has a pleasantly sweet, apple-like flavor. The flavonoids in chamomile bind to receptors in the brain that dampen overactivity and promote calm. Chamomile also contains the compound apigenin, which reduces anxiety by binding to specific GABA receptors in the brain. This produces a mild sedative effect similar to anti-anxiety medications. Furthermore, chamomile relieves muscle spasms and tension by blocking calcium channels that stimulate contraction. All these actions translate to noticeable relaxation of both mind and body.

Lavender comes from another member of the Asteraceae family, Lavandula angustifolia. The purple flowers are where lavender gets its familiar fragrance, which aromatherapists describe as floral, herbaceous, and slightly fruity. Lavender contains antioxidant polyphenols like rosmarinic acid that curb anxiety not only through scent but also through direct anti-anxiety actions in the brain. Like chamomile, lavender modulates GABA neurotransmission and levels of serotonin, dopamine, and norepinephrine - brain chemicals that regulate mood and stress response. Human studies confirm lavender's ability to reduce tension, irritability, and restlessness while improving sleep quality.

Together, chamomile and lavender make an optimal pairing for relaxing tension relief. Chamomile quiets the nerves while lavender soothes and uplifts the spirit. The beauty of this blend is its mildness and safety. Unlike prescription sedatives and anxiety drugs, chamomile and lavender are non-habit forming and generally don't cause drowsiness. Enjoy a cup in the afternoon or evening to gently unwind. It's equally soothing before bed to ease into sleep.

To brew a tension tamer tea, steep 2 teaspoons of dried chamomile flowers and 1 teaspoon of dried lavender buds in a cup of hot (not boiling) water for 5 to 7 minutes. Covering the cup while steeping preserves the volatile aromatics. The strength can be adjusted to taste. Add a drizzle of honey, a squeeze of lemon, or a sprinkle of dried rose petals to complement the floral flavors. Sip slowly, close your eyes, and feel the worries of the day start to evaporate.

Anxiety, stress, and overwhelm are unfortunately inevitable parts of life. However, herbs like chamomile and lavender provide natural ways to help break free from that tension when we start to feel tangled up in knots. With a warm cup of this soothing blend, take a mini-vacation whenever you need to relax and rebalance. Let the sweet floral aromas and mellow bittersweet taste transport you to a peaceful state of mind.

Calming Catnip and Passionflower Blend

Feeling stressed and anxious? Let nature help you chill out with a relaxing cup of catnip and passionflower tea. Far from being just for felines, the herb catnip has a long history of use as a mild sedative for humans. When blended with passionflower, known for easing anxiety and insomnia, it makes a tasty calming brew. Read on to learn all about this purr-fectly soothing combo.

Nepeta cataria is the formal name for the herb commonly known as catnip. Native to Europe and parts of Asia, it has been naturalized in North America and grows wild in some areas. Often seen growing along roads or at the edge of wooded areas, catnip is a stout perennial herb of the mint family, with serrated heart-shaped leaves and small white or lavender flowers. Interestingly, cats' extreme attraction to catnip is triggered by substances called nepetalactone found in the leaves and stems, but these compounds do not affect humans in the same way. We experience catnip's mild sedative effects. Dried catnip makes a pleasantly minty, citrusy tea on its own, but blending with other herbs enhances its calming qualities.

Passionflower, or Passiflora incarnata, perfectly complements catnip for an anxiety-busting brew. It too grows wild throughout North America, recognizable by its unique blooms with ornate radial filaments. Various Native American tribes traditionally used passionflower as a general calming remedy and sleep aid. Today, it is an approved over-the-counter sedative in Europe. Clinical research suggests passion flower increases levels of the neurotransmitter gamma-aminobutyric acid (GABA) in the brain. GABA helps quiet nervous system activity, reducing anxiety, irritability, and worry. The flavonoids in passionflower also have a benzodiazepine-like action on GABA receptors, meaning they bind to the same sites as prescription anti-anxiety drugs. No wonder Passionflower eases away feelings of tension and agitation!

By combining catnip and passionflower, their mild sedative actions complement each other. Catnip's active compounds nepetalactone, citral, and citronellal, work with passion flowers GABA-boosting flavonoids for a synergistic anti-anxiety effect. More than the sum of their parts, this dynamic duo relaxes the mind and body from the inside out. Both herbs have an extensive history of use and safety, with no risk of habit formation. Simply put, they induce tranquility the natural way.

Want to make a cup of calming catnip and passionflower tea? Simply add 1-2 teaspoons each of the dried herbs to 8 ounces of hot water and steep for 5 to 10 minutes. Sweetening with a bit of honey enhances the mild, grassy flavor. Sipping this brew slowly in the evening helps unwind before bedtime. It's also perfect for taking the edge off any time stress starts to creep up during your day. The tea can be enjoyed either hot or iced. For best results, cover the cup while steeping to retain the herbs beneficial volatile oils.

In our hectic modern world, taking intentional relaxation breaks is crucial for health and well-being. Instead of reaching for pharmaceutical sedatives, turn to the gentle plants catnip and passionflower for natural relief from pent up tension. Keep a supply of the dried herbs on hand for brewing comforting cups of tea when life leaves you feeling frazzled. The soothing experience of preparing and savoring this herbal infusion lets you collect yourself and find your calm center. Discover the power of plants to bring balance and solace whenever you need it.

Sleepytime - Valerian and Ashwagandha

Do you regularly toss and turn, struggling to fall asleep and stay asleep? Insomnia can leave you utterly exhausted yet frustratingly wide awake when you want so desperately to rest. Racing thoughts, anxiety, everyday stresses, underlying health issues, and side effects from medications are just some reasons sleep may elude you. Luckily, herbs that gently sedate and relax the nervous system can help pave the way for deep, rejuvenating slumber. Enter valerian and ashwagandha - two of nature's most renowned sleep aids. Combined into one potent nighttime tea, they can work wonders to improve your sleep quality naturally.

Valerian is a perennial flowering plant indigenous to Europe and parts of Asia. With clusters of sweetly scented white or pink flowers, valerian thrives along roadsides and drier grasslands. The root is the medicinal part of the plant, prized for its sedative properties. Valerian extract has been used for centuries as a sleep aid and anxiety reliever. Compounds called valerenic acids and valeranone block excessive activity in the nervous system by increasing GABA levels and binding to GABA receptors. This has a calming, sedative effect much like prescription sleeping pills. However, valerian is not addictive and does not cause morning grogginess like some pharmaceutical sleep aids.

Ashwagandha, also known as Indian ginseng or winter cherry, is an important herb in Ayurvedic healing traditions. The small shrub bears red berries and has been used for over 3,000 years to boost vitality and relieve stress. With potent adaptogenic and calming properties, ashwagandha is excellent for lowering cortisol and dialing down the nervous system when sleep escapes you. Key bioactive compounds called withanolides are responsible for ashwagandha's anti-anxiety, anti-stress benefits. It also increases GABA levels while reducing excitatory neurotransmissions. This combination of actions promotes deeper, more restorative sleep.

By pairing valerian's sedative properties with ashwagandha's adaptogenic balancing effects, the two herbs complement each other beautifully. Valerian helps the body ease into drowsiness while ashwagandha alleviates the mind-racing, restless thoughts that often accompany insomnia. Steep 1-2 teaspoons each of dried valerian root and ashwagandha root powder in a cup of hot water for 10 minutes. Sweeten with honey if desired. Sip an hour before bedtime for best results. Some people find the earthy, slightly bitter taste of valerian unpleasant, so adding lemon, ginger, mint, or other herbs helps mellow the flavor. Also consider taking in capsule form if the taste is unappealing.

Give this Sleepytime tea blend a try if you regularly struggle with falling or staying asleep. Over time, valerian and ashwagandha work to regulate your sleep cycle so you can effortlessly drift off to sleep and wake refreshed. As nervous system tonics, they impart healthy long term benefits beyond just the immediate sedative effects. Your mind, body, and mood will thank you for the healing gift of deep sleep aided by nature's remedies. You may find yourself eagerly looking forward to sipping a steamy cup of Sleepytime tea as you wind down each evening, knowing restful slumber awaits.

De-Stress Digestif - Fennel and Lemon Balm

Feeling stressed out, anxious, and overwhelmed? As much as we try to avoid it, nearly everyone experiences these tense feelings at times. Pressure from work, family obligations, finances, health issues, and current events winds us up and frays our nerves. Even small daily annoyances can accumulate and push our stress response into overdrive. This wreaks havoc on both physical and mental health. While we can't eliminate stressors, we can actively calm our nervous system to prevent heading into meltdown mode. Sipping relaxing herbal tea is one of the most pleasant ways to hit the reset button when you're all wound up. One excellent blend for soothing stress combines fennel and lemon balm - two herbs with centuries-old use for reducing anxiety and settling the stomach.

Fennel is a hardy perennial that thrives throughout temperate regions across the globe. With feathery fronds and yellow flowers, it bears aromatic seeds used as a spice and medicine. Folk healers have utilized fennel to calm the gut and nervous system since ancient times. Studies confirm that compounds like anethole, limonene, and quercetin give fennel anti-anxiety properties. Anethole in particular exhibits anti-stress activity by lowering cortisol levels. Anethole and limonene also relax intestinal muscles for relief from the stomach upset that often accompanies anxiety. Who knew fennel offered such wide-ranging benefits beyond seasoning foods?

Pairing fennel with lemon balm makes for a soothing brew to sip when you're stressed and need to decompress. Melissa officinalis is the scientific name for this hardy herb from the mint family. With its lemony aroma and flavor, lemon balm has a long history of use for reducing anxiety, soothing the stomach, and lifting mood. It contains potent plant compounds like rosmarinic acid, luteolin, and triterpenes that work on GABA receptors and other brain signaling pathways involved in the stress response. In short, lemon balm is a clinically proven chill pill without the side effects of Rx tranquilizers.

Brew a cup using 1 teaspoon each of dried, crushed fennel seed and dried lemon balm leaves steeped for 5 to 10 minutes in hot water. The flavors meld together nicely, with fennel's light anise taste complementing the bright lemon notes. Add a spoonful of honey if desired. Slowly sipping this aromatic tea lets your mind decompress as your digestive system smooths out. Fennel and lemon balm work synergistically to promote a sense of tranquility from the inside out. No longer tense and anxious, you'll feel your body relax and your typical good humor return.

We all face times when responsibilities, struggles, and the frenetic pace of life leave us tied up in knots. Turn to fennel and lemon balm for a natural way to settle your stomach, ease anxiety, and regain calm composure. Keep the dried herbs on hand and brew a cup as needed whenever you're feeling overwhelmed and jittery. The comfort of savoring this medicinal tea lets you proactively care for your nervous system and restore peace of mind.

Anxiety Antidote - CBD and L-Theanine

Feel like your anxiety has the upper hand these days? You're not alone. Anxiety disorders are pervasive in modern society, with an estimated 40 million American adults suffering from anxiety each year. Constant worrying, rumination, tension, panic attacks, and feeling overwhelmed by daily responsibilities are completely exhausting, not to mention detrimental to your physical health. Pharmaceutical medications like benzodiazepines commonly prescribed for anxiety, unfortunately, come with side effects and risk of dependence. For a natural alternative without the downsides, consider sipping CBD and L-theanine tea when anxiety strikes. These two plant-based compounds work synergistically to calm nerves and quiet the mind without sedation or addiction potential.

You may have heard about cannabidiol, better known as CBD, as a treatment for epilepsy, pain, and other health conditions. CBD is a compound abundant in cannabis and hemp plants but lacks the psychoactive effects of THC. Our bodies actually produce their own endogenous cannabinoids as part of the endocannabinoid system that regulates mood, pain, appetite, and more. Plant-derived CBD supports this regulatory system for wide-ranging therapeutic benefits. For anxiety sufferers, CBD ingestion has a clinically proven calming effect by changing serotonin signals in the brain and reducing excitation in the nervous system. Numerous studies confirm CBD's effectiveness for reducing stress, anxiety, and even social anxiety disorder with no adverse side effects.

Pairing CBD with L-theanine magnifies these anxiolytic benefits. L-theanine is an amino acid found primarily in tea leaves that produces feelings of tranquility. It binds to brain receptors for the neurotransmitter glutamate and changes signaling patterns to curb excitatory neurotransmission. At the same time, L-theanine boosts alpha waves in the brain linked to relaxed mental focus. Its ability to take the edge off anxious feelings makes it the perfect complement to CBD. Combining these two compounds allows CBD to maximize anti-anxiety benefits while L-theanine smoothes out any potential side effects like drowsiness.

Anxiety Antidote - CBD and L-Theanine

Feel like your anxiety has the upper hand these days? You're not alone. Anxiety disorders are pervasive in modern society, with an estimated 40 million American adults suffering from anxiety each year. Constant worrying, rumination, tension, panic attacks, and feeling overwhelmed by daily responsibilities are completely exhausting, not to mention detrimental to your physical health. Pharmaceutical medications like benzodiazepines commonly prescribed for anxiety, unfortunately, come with side effects and risk of dependence. For a natural alternative without the downsides, consider sipping CBD and L-theanine tea when anxiety strikes. These two plant-based compounds work synergistically to calm nerves and quiet the mind without sedation or addiction potential.

You may have heard about cannabidiol, better known as CBD, as a treatment for epilepsy, pain, and other health conditions. CBD is a compound abundant in cannabis and hemp plants but lacks the psychoactive effects of THC. Our bodies actually produce their own endogenous cannabinoids as part of the endocannabinoid system that regulates mood, pain, appetite, and more. Plant-derived CBD supports this regulatory system for wide-ranging therapeutic benefits. For anxiety sufferers, CBD ingestion has a clinically proven calming effect by changing serotonin signals in the brain and reducing excitation in the nervous system. Numerous studies confirm CBD's effectiveness for reducing stress, anxiety, and even social anxiety disorder with no adverse side effects.

Pairing CBD with L-theanine magnifies these anxiolytic benefits. L-theanine is an amino acid found primarily in tea leaves that produces feelings of tranquility. It binds to brain receptors for the neurotransmitter glutamate and changes signaling patterns to curb excitatory neurotransmission. At the same time, L-theanine boosts alpha waves in the brain linked to relaxed mental focus. Its ability to take the edge off anxious feelings makes it the perfect complement to CBD. Combining these two compounds allows CBD to maximize anti-anxiety benefits while L-theanine smoothes out any potential side effects like drowsiness.

The simplest method is buying ready-made CBD and L-theanine tea bags, which provide pre-measured quantities of both compounds. Otherwise, add a dropper full of liquid CBD extract and 200mg L-theanine powder to hot water and mix well. Start with a low CBD dose like 10-15mg and increase slowly as needed. The earthy, botanical flavors blend smoothly. Drink whenever you feel anxiety building for relief within 30-60 minutes. Over time, consistency helps rebalance brain chemistry for an overall reduction in chronic anxiety.

Rather than popping anti-anxiety medications, look to nature for safe, effective solutions. This CBD and L-theanine tea combo nourishes your endocannabinoid system and keeps neurotransmissions cool, calm, and collected. Treat yourself to this soothing tea whenever you feel your thoughts spiraling out of control. It allows you to step back from the chaos of anxious minds and find your inner stillness.

Sencha Green Tea

Do you start each day feeling frazzled, anxious, and overwhelmed? Or maybe mental tension starts to build in the afternoons, making it hard to stay focused at work. Feeling constantly relaxed and clear-headed can be a challenge in our hectic modern lives. Stress is simply unavoidable. Luckily, certain teas have natural calming and focus-enhancing effects that can help you find your zen. Japanese sencha green tea is a particularly wonderful choice for its soothing yet energizing qualities.

Sencha occupies a special place among Japanese green teas. It has a vegetal, umami flavor and high concentrations of bioactive compounds that provide both mental clarity and tranquil relaxation. This makes it a uniquely soothing beverage for chaotic times. Read on to learn all about Sencha and how sipping this green tea regularly benefits your mind-body balance.

Production Process

All tea comes from the leaves of Camellia sinensis, and differences in processing give each style its signature flavors and benefits. For Japanese sencha green tea, the leaves are steamed, rolled, and dried immediately after harvest. Minimal processing preserves Sencha's fresh flavor and high antioxidant content compared to other teas. The name sencha translates to "simmered tea" in Japanese, describing the key steaming step. This destroys enzymes that would otherwise oxidize and degrade valuable catechins, the main antioxidants in green tea.

Sencha should not be confused with matcha, a fine powdered green tea used in the traditional tea ceremony. While matcha contains more total catechins, sencha has a more complex catechin profile that some studies suggest provides greater cognitive benefits. The largest catechin fraction is EGCG, a potent antioxidant that readily crosses the blood-brain barrier. Along with boosting brain function, EGCG has anti-anxiety effects by modulating neurotransmitters and hormones involved in the stress response.

Taste and Aroma

The flavor of sencha ranges from vegetal grassy to subtly sweet. High-quality sencha has an umami or oceanic savoriness, while lower grades may taste overly grassy or bitter. The aroma is fresh and green with notes of seaweed, cut grass, spinach, and asparagus. Infusing sencha with cooler water around 160°F preserves sweetness, while hotter temperatures extract more vegetal, oceanic flavors. Green tea's natural bitterness means sencha is often enjoyed plain without milk or sweetener, allowing its pure flavor to shine.

How Sencha Calms and Relaxes

Sencha's relaxing yet clarifying effect on the mind and body is largely attributed to its caffeine and L-theanine content. All true teas contain some caffeine, but Sencha's lower oxidation means more caffeine remains intact versus black teas. The caffeine provides a gentle energizing lift without overstimulating. L-theanine, an amino acid in tea leaves, has anti-stress benefits by increasing alpha brain waves associated with relaxed focus. It also changes neurotransmitter levels in the brain for mood stabilization. The symbiotic combination of caffeine and L-theanine in sencha produces a calm, alert state free of jitteriness.

Additionally, sencha's high antioxidant content scavenges damaging free radicals caused by a stressful environment and poor diet. Oxidative stress contributes to anxiety, fatigue, poor immunity, and low mood. The polyphenols in sencha tea combat that internal stress damage, allowing your body and mind to function at their best. Improved circulation from drinking sencha also increases oxygen and nutrient flow to the brain. Taken together, sencha green tea provides both immediate pleasure and long-term benefits that enhance mental resilience.

Brewing Sencha Tea

To brew sencha, use 2-3 grams of leaves per 6 ounces of water heated to 160-180°F. Steeping at lower temperatures helps avoid bitterness while high temperatures can extract astringent tannins. Steep 1-2 minutes for the first infusion, adding 15-30 seconds for subsequent infusions. Some sencha can sustain up to five infusions, increasing the value of your tea leaves. Always brew in a ceramic or glass teapot for the best flavor. Let the pale greenish infusion cool slightly before enjoying its sublime taste and aroma. Sip slowly over a period of quiet relaxation and reflection.

Drinking sencha tea is part of an overall lifestyle that prizes quality over quantity, community, and harmonious living. Beyond the antioxidants and brain-boosting compounds, sencha represents a break from constant stimulation and distraction. The practice of preparing, appreciating, and mindfully sipping sencha instills a sense of inner calm. Incorporate sencha into your daily routine for clarity, focus, and tranquility in the midst of life's chaos.

Chapter 4

Herbal Teas for Soothing Digestion

Herbal teas have been used for centuries to help soothe digestive upsets and promote overall digestive health. The medicinal compounds in herbs can provide relief from symptoms like nausea, gas, bloating, stomach pain, and indigestion. Sipping on a comforting cup of tea made from gut-friendly herbs can be a tasty way to find belly comfort when digestive troubles flare up.

Certain herbs contain compounds that help relax gastrointestinal muscles, reduce inflammation, stimulate bile flow, and act as prebiotics to feed healthy gut bacteria. Other herbs contain antioxidants, antispasmodic, and pain-relieving properties ideal for calming an unhappy belly. Traditional herbal teas made from roots, seeds, leaves, fruits, and flowers from plants like ginger, peppermint, chamomile, and fennel can be extremely effective at easing all kinds of digestive woes.

Belly Comfort: Peppermint and Ginger

When your stomach just feels off and your belly needs a little TLC, turning to a cup of peppermint and ginger tea can help relax digestive muscles, reduce inflammation and gas, and provide soothing comfort. Studies show this powerful herb duo is highly effective at relieving abdominal pain, distension, and cramping and improving overall gastric motility.

The menthol in peppermint has analgesic, invigorating, and cooling properties that provide a calming sensation throughout the intestines. Peppermint helps relax intestinal smooth muscle to relieve painful spasms, cramping, and urgency associated with irritable bowel syndrome (IBS). The volatile oils in peppermint also have carminative effects to help reduce bloating, gas, and flatulence through relaxation of the esophageal sphincter.

Ginger contains potent anti-inflammatory compounds called gingerols that inhibit the production of inflammatory prostaglandins to ease stomach discomfort. Ginger helps speed up gastric emptying by increasing motility, while also preventing motion sickness, nausea, and vomiting. This zesty root warms and stimulates digestion to relieve bloating, cramping, diarrhea, and constipation.

Simmer 1-2 teaspoons of freshly grated ginger root and a handful of peppermint leaves in hot water for 10 minutes to extract the therapeutic compounds. Drink this aroma-therapeutic tea when experiencing generalized abdominal discomfort, pain, cramping or slow digestion. The spicy-cool combination of ginger and mint will help relax your belly while reducing inflammation for fast relief.

Bloat Buster: Fennel, Cardamom, and Cinnamon

Bloating is one of the most common and uncomfortable digestive issues. Gas buildup from trouble digesting certain foods can leave the belly distended and painful. Herbal teas made with carminative herbs that help expel intestinal gas can provide quick relief for bloated bellies.

Fennel seeds contain estragole, fenchone, and anethole - compounds that help relax smooth muscle in the digestive tract to release trapped gas and reduce bloating. Fennel also boosts bile production to improve fat digestion and prevent gas production from undigested fats.

Cardamom pods contain cineole and limonene - compounds that have antispasmodic effects on the gastrointestinal tract to relieve gas pains and cramping. Cardamom also increases gastric secretions like bile and acids to improve digestion and prevent gas-causing fermentation.

Cinnamon is rich in antioxidants and essential oils that provide anti-inflammatory, antispasmodic benefits to soothe intestinal muscle spasms and aid digestion. Cinnamon also slows gastric emptying to prevent gas caused by eating too quickly.

For fast relief from a bloated, gassy belly, steep 1-2 teaspoons each of fennel seeds, cardamom pods, and cinnamon sticks in hot water for 10-15 minutes. The aromatic oils and phytochemicals will work quickly to relax the gut, dispel gas, and relieve abdominal pressure and discomfort. Drink a few cups of this tea daily when experiencing frequent bloating.

Nausea No More: Ginger, Licorice, and Slippery Elm

Nausea is one of the worst feelings when you have an upset stomach. Thankfully, certain herbal teas can help quickly calm waves of nausea for relief when you need it most. A soothing combination of ginger, licorice root, and slippery elm makes a therapeutic tea for settling queasiness.

Ginger is arguably the most effective herb for treating nausea. Compounds called gingerols and shogaols exert anti-emetic effects by blocking serotonin receptors to prevent triggering the vomit reflex. Hot or cold ginger tea can quickly calm nausea from motion sickness, pregnancy, chemotherapy drugs or gastrointestinal issues.

Licorice root contains triterpenoids like glycyrrhizin that help coat and protect the stomach lining to prevent nausea triggered by excess stomach acid. Licorice is also naturally sweet, which can help overcome nausea caused by hunger or low blood sugar.

Slippery elm forms a mucilaginous gel when mixed with water that helps coat and soothe the digestive tract to ease nausea, reflux, and vomiting. The antioxidants in slippery elm also help reduce inflammation associated with nausea and poor digestion.

For fast relief from an unsettled, queasy stomach, steep 1-inch ginger root, 1 teaspoon licorice root, and 1 teaspoon slippery elm bark in hot water for 10 minutes. Sip slowly, allowing the mucilaginous brew to thoroughly coat the digestive tract and ease stomach upset. Drink 1-3 cups daily as needed for nausea relief.

Heartburn Helper: Chamomile, Marshmallow Root, and Meadowsweet

The burning discomfort caused by acid reflux can make enjoying meals unpleasant. Herbal teas made from plants like chamomile, marshmallow root, and meadowsweet can help provide relief from the painful effects of excess stomach acid.

Chamomile contains apigenin, a natural anti-inflammatory flavonoid that helps reduce inflammation in the esophagus caused by stomach acid backing up through a weakened esophageal sphincter. The soothing antioxidants in chamomile also decrease histamine production to prevent acid secretion.

Marshmallow root is a demulcent herb that forms a protective mucilage when steeped in hot water that adheres to mucous membranes and helps create a barrier against stomach acid. This helps reduce inflammation and discomfort from reflux. The mucilage also helps coat and heal damaged tissues.

Meadowsweet contains salicylates and polyphenols that help suppress stomach acid production and reduce inflammation. Meadowsweet increases mucus secretions in the stomach, building up a barrier against erosive acid. The herb also has natural antacid effects to help neutralize excess acid.

For soothing relief from the burning pain of acid reflux, steep 2 teaspoons of dried chamomile flowers, marshmallow root, and meadowsweet leaves in hot water for 10 minutes. Drink after meals to prevent painful flare-ups and reduce acid damage to the esophagus. This healing tea will help strengthen your lower esophageal sphincter and rebuild damaged tissue.

Detox Digestif: Dandelion, Milk Thistle, and Peppermint

Indulging in heavy comfort foods can leave you feeling sluggish and backed up. Herbal teas made with detoxifying herbs like dandelion, milk thistle, and peppermint can help get things moving again by stimulating digestion and supporting healthy liver function.

Dandelion roots and leaves contain inulin, a prebiotic fiber that feeds probiotics to support healthy gut flora. The choline in dandelion also helps stimulate bile production to improve fat digestion and elimination. Dandelion has a mild laxative effect to relieve constipation.

Milk thistle contains silymarin, an antioxidant compound that protects liver cells from damage while stimulating regeneration and protein synthesis. This helps improve the liver's ability to filter toxins and produce bile for better digestion and detoxification.

Peppermint contains menthol, a volatile oil that relaxes intestinal muscles to relieve spasms and stimulates the flow of bile from the liver and gallbladder. This helps improve digestion and elimination of waste through increased bile flow.

For an herbal cleanse after heavy eating, steep 2 teaspoons each of dandelion root, milk thistle seeds, and peppermint leaves in hot water for 10 minutes. Drink 1-2 cups in the morning and evening to support healthy digestion, liver function, and regular bowel movements for improved detoxification. This blend will get your digestive system moving smoothly again.

Prebiotic Tummy Tamer: Chicory Root and Star Anise

Having enough healthy gut flora is essential for proper digestion and preventing issues like gas, bloating, and indigestion. Prebiotic herbs like chicory root and star anise can help feed and flourish populations of beneficial bacteria for a happy belly.

Chicory root is a great source of inulin, a prebiotic fiber that passes undigested through the upper GI tract and feeds bacteria like Bifidobacterium and Lactobacillus species in the colon. This helps boost populations of bacteria that promote proper digestion, nutrient absorption, and regularity.

Star anise contains antioxidant flavonoids like quercetin that have antibacterial effects against harmful pathogens like E.coli and Candida while leaving populations of beneficial flora intact. This helps prevent an imbalance between good and bad bacteria.

Steeping chicory root and star anise create a tea rich in prebiotics for nourishing healthy gut flora and antioxidants to inhibit bad bacteria overgrowth. For improved digestion from a thriving microbiome, steep 2 teaspoons each of chicory root and star anise pods in hot water for 10-15 minutes. Drink 1-2 cups daily to keep digestive woes at bay.

Herbal teas are an easy, effective way to find relief from many minor to moderate digestive complaints. The medicinal compounds in herbs like peppermint, ginger, chamomile, fennel, and dandelion can help relax gastrointestinal muscles, reduce inflammation, stimulate digestion, and support detoxification for improved comfort and function. Drinking teas made from these gut-soothing plants can provide natural relief without harsh side effects. Explore incorporating more of these delicious botanical brews into your daily routine for optimal digestive wellness.

More Herbal Teas for Digestive Wellness

In the vast world of botanical remedies, there are countless herbs that can be brewed into teas to help provide relief for all kinds of digestive troubles. Beyond classic digestive aids like ginger, chamomile, and peppermint, there are many more healing herbs to discover that can ease stomach woes ranging from constipation to diarrhea.

Medicinal plants contain a diverse array of phytochemicals and aromatic compounds that make them highly effective at addressing the root causes of digestion issues. Soothing herbs like marshmallow and licorice can reduce inflammation in the GI tract. Antispasmodic herbs such as fennel and lemon balm can relax cramping and spasms. Carminative herbs like cinnamon and cardamom help expel gas. Demulcent herbs like slippery elm and marshmallows form protective mucilage. Prebiotics in plants like chicory feed good bacteria.

Natural Relief for Constipation

Being backed up and unable to eliminate waste comfortably can make anyone feel lousy. Thankfully there are many herbal remedies that can get things moving again and provide natural relief from constipation. Specific herbs contain compounds and fibers that help stimulate contractions, draw water into the colon to soften stools, and support healthy gut motility and elimination.

Senna - This herb contains anthraquinone glycosides that stimulate contractions in the colon to trigger bowel movements. Senna promotes the secretion of fluid into the intestines to help soften and move along hard dry stools. Start with low doses as senna can cause cramping in high amounts.

Psyllium - The mucilaginous fiber in psyllium husks absorbs water and swells up to add bulk and moisture to stools. This helps stimulate peristalsis and makes elimination easier and more comfortable. Psyllium also acts as a prebiotic to feed healthy gut flora.

Aloe Vera - Compounds like aloin and barbaloin give aloe vera leaf its laxative effects by stimulating colon contractions and increasing intestinal water content to make stools softer. Aloe helps improve regularity and ease constipation related to irritable bowel syndrome.

Triphala - This Ayurvedic blend contains three dried fruits - amalaki, bibhitaki, and haritaki - that work together to stimulate gentle contractions of the gastrointestinal tract. Triphala also contains antioxidants that support healthy digestion and elimination.

Dandelion - Inulin fiber and bitter compounds called taraxacin and taracerin in dandelion promote bile secretion and act as a mild laxative to increase intestinal motility and stimulate contractions. This aids in more regular bowel movements.

To help get things moving, try combining 1 part senna, 1 part psyllium husks, 1 part aloe vera, ½ part Triphala powder, and ½ part dandelion root. Steep 1-2 teaspoons of the herb blend in boiling water for 10 minutes. Drink once daily preferably in the morning for relief from constipation. Be sure to also drink plenty of fluids.

Soothing an Upset Stomach and Diarrhea

Stomach bugs, food poisoning and intestinal infections can all cause uncomfortable diarrhea, abdominal cramping, and urgency. Herbal teas made with plants containing tannins, mucilage, and antioxidants can help soothe inflammation, reduce spasms, and firm up loose stools for relief from diarrhea.

Blackberry Leaf - This herb is rich in astringent tannins that help constrict intestinal tissues and tighten loose stools. Blackberry leaf also reduces inflammation and contains antioxidants that fight bacteria overgrowth causing diarrhea.

Marshmallow Root - The mucilage in marshmallow root coats, soothes, and protects irritated intestinal tissues. This helps reduce inflammation and alleviate cramps, spasms, and discomfort from diarrhea or IBS.

Agrimony - In addition to its astringent tannins, agrimony also contains analgesic and antispasmodic compounds that help relieve cramps, urgent diarrhea, and other gastric distress symptoms.

Cinnamon - The essential oils and tannins in cinnamon bark have an astringent effect to firm up loose stools and slow motility to prevent urgent diarrhea. Cinnamon also reduces inflammation and fights harmful bacteria.

Ginger - Gingerols and other compounds in ginger suppress muscle spasms and slow motility to reduce episodes of cramping and diarrhea. Ginger also decreases inflammation and nausea.

For relief from urgent, frequent diarrhea, brew a tea with 1 tablespoon each of blackberry leaf, marshmallow root, agrimony, and cinnamon chips plus 1 teaspoon of freshly grated ginger. Steep in boiling water for 10-15 minutes and drink up to 3 times daily to soothe diarrhea. Be sure to also replenish fluids and electrolytes.

Settling Indigestion and Heartburn

That burning pain rising from the stomach after meals can signal indigestion, or in more severe cases, gastroesophageal reflux disease (GERD). Herbal teas can help settle the stomach, reduce inflammation and acid production, and heal damaged tissues.

Licorice Root - Compounds in licorice-like glycyrrhizin help protect the stomach lining from acid irritation and inhibit the secretion of gastric acids and pepsin to prevent reflux. Licorice also increases mucus.

Marshmallow Root - The mucilaginous compounds in marshmallow root coat and soothe tissues damaged by excess acid. This helps reduce inflammation and heal ulceration in the esophagus from reflux.

Slippery Elm - Like marshmallows, slippery elm contains mucilage that adheres to the esophageal lining to shield it from erosion from stomach acid. Slippery elm also helps neutralize acids.

Meadowsweet - Meadowsweet contains anti-inflammatory salicylates similar to aspirin that help suppress excess acid secretion associated with heartburn and gastritis.

Calendula - Soothing anti-inflammatory flavonoids found in calendula flowers help accelerate the healing process and repair tissue damage caused by excess stomach acids.

For relief from the pain and discomfort of heartburn and indigestion, steep 1 tablespoon each of licorice root, marshmallow root, slippery elm, meadowsweet, and calendula in hot water. Drink 30 minutes before meals to build up mucilage and after meals to coat and protect tissues from acids.

Relieving Nausea and Loss of Appetite

Persistent feelings of nausea can prevent proper food intake and lead to weight loss and nutritional deficits. Sipping on teas made with anti-emetic and stomach-soothing herbs can help overcome nausea while stimulating appetite.

Herbal Teas for Optimal Digestive Wellness

Achieving an optimally functioning digestive system is essential to overall health and vitality. Herbal teas offer a tasty, aromatic way to nourish every aspect of your gastrointestinal tract. Certain herbs excel at soothing inflammation, destroying pathogens, stimulating digestion, relaxing intestinal muscles, supporting healthy gut flora, and assisting in regular elimination.

Discover more gut-friendly teas to incorporate into your daily routine for improved nutrient absorption, easier elimination, relief from discomfort, and protection from disease. Drink your way to robust digestive wellness with these research-backed botanical brews.

Relaxing Intestinal Spasms and Colic

Painful spasms and cramping in the intestines can make life miserable. Antispasmodic herbs contain compounds that help relax smooth muscle tissue in the gastrointestinal tract to provide relief from muscle tightness and colicky contractions.

Chamomile - Apigenin and other natural compounds give chamomile anti-inflammatory and antispasmodic properties that alleviate intestinal cramping related to IBS, colic, ulcers, and more.

Peppermint - Menthol in peppermint relaxes intestinal muscles and eases spastic contractions to reduce cramping from gas pains, bloating, constipation, and diarrhea.

Wild Yam - Steroidal saponins called diosgenin in wild yam have antispasmodic effects on smooth muscles in the GI tract to relieve colic, menstrual cramps, and nerve pain.

Fennel - Anethole, estragole, and other compounds in fennel seeds block muscle spasms in the intestines and suppress gastrointestinal motility to ease colic and cramping.

Catnip - Nepetalactone gives catnip its ability to settle the stomach by reducing gastric acid secretion and relaxing intestinal muscles to relieve painful cramps and spasms.

For natural cramp relief, steep 2 teaspoons each of dried chamomile, peppermint leaves, wild yam, fennel seeds, and catnip in hot water for 10 minutes. Drink as needed to relieve acute intestinal spasms and prevent recurring colicky pains.

Improving Digestion and Nutrient Absorption

Sluggish digestion can lead to gas, bloating, and nutritional deficiencies. Herbal remedies known as digestifs contain compounds that stimulate digestion to boost the assimilation of nutrients from food.

Ginger - Gingerols speed up the movement of food through the GI tract and increase the production of saliva, bile, and gastric juices to improve digestion and emptying of the stomach.

Black Pepper - Piperine enhances the bioavailability of nutrients by stimulating gastric enzymes and improving the transportation of amino acids across the intestinal lining.

Gentian - Bitter compounds like gentiopicrin prompt increased bile and saliva production while stimulating gastric emptying to aid digestion, especially of fats.

Fennel - Estragole, fenchone, and other phytochemicals in fennel promote the secretion of digestive enzymes and bile to break down food and improve mineral absorption.

Cardamom - 1,8-Cineole and other aromatic compounds boost bile production and increase gastric secretions like acids and enzymes for more efficient digestion.

For improved digestion and nutrient absorption, combine 2 teaspoons each of grated ginger, crushed black peppercorns, dried gentian root, fennel seeds, and ground cardamom. Steep in hot water for 10-15 minutes before drinking 30 minutes before meals.

Combating Hemorrhoids

Inflamed veins in and around the anus and lower rectum can cause painful, itchy hemorrhoids. Astringent herbal teas can help tighten tissues, reduce swelling, and improve circulation to alleviate hemorrhoid misery.

Witch Hazel - Tannins in witch hazel leaves constrict veins and shrink swollen, inflamed tissues providing cooling relief from irritation, burning, and itching.

Bilberry - Potent antioxidants called anthocyanosides to strengthen blood vessel walls and improve circulation in veins to reduce hemorrhoid flare-ups.

White Oak - Like witch hazel, white oak bark is rich in tannins that tighten vascular tissues to decrease swelling of varicose veins causing hemorrhoids.

Horse Chestnut - Aescin and other anti-inflammatory compounds found in horse chestnut seeds help tone vein walls, reduce swelling, and improve circulation to affected areas.

Butcher's Broom - Ruscogenins and saponins in butcher's broom rhizome exhibit mild vasoconstrictor effects to reduce inflammation and strengthen capillaries.

For relief from the discomfort of enlarged, inflamed hemorrhoids steep 3 tablespoons of dried witch hazel leaves, 1 tablespoon of bilberry leaves, 2 teaspoons white oak bark, 1 teaspoon horse chestnut, and 1/2 teaspoon butcher's broom in hot water for 10 minutes. Drink up to 3 times daily.

Cleansing the Colon and Improving Regularity

Keeping your colon clean and free of waste buildup is key for healthy elimination and preventing toxicity. Herbs like senna, psyllium, and aloe vera act as colon cleansers and natural laxatives.

Senna- Anthraquinone glycosides in senna stimulate intestinal contractions to push out waste and clear obstructions. This provides relief from constipation.

Psyllium- Fibrous husks swell with water to add bulk to stools, making elimination easier. Psyllium also acts as a prebiotic to feed healthy bacteria.

Aloe Vera- Compounds like aloin and barbaloin give aloe vera its gentle laxative effect by softening stools and inducing bowel movements.

Triphala- This traditional Ayurvedic blend of three dried fruits gently stimulates colonic motility to improve regularity without griping or pain.

Dandelion- Chicoric acid, inulin fiber, and bitter compounds make dandelion root a mild laxative to increase bile flow and intestinal contractions.

For a natural colon cleanse, combine 2 parts psyllium husks, 1 part senna leaves, 1 part aloe vera gel, ½ part Triphala powder, and ½ part dandelion root. Steep 1-2 teaspoons in hot water and drink daily to support healthy elimination.

Soothe Ulcers, Gastritis, and GERD

Painful inflammation in the stomach or esophagus caused by H. pylori bacteria or excess stomach acid can disrupt eating and damage tissues. Herbal teas can help heal these digestive ailments.

Marshmallow Root- Mucilaginous compounds coat, soothe and protect tissues from excess acid and enzymes allowing ulcers and erosion to heal.

Slippery Elm- Like marshmallows, slippery elm bark contains mucilage that adheres to the stomach lining to shield it from irritation and inflammation.

Licorice Root- Triterpenoids like glycyrrhizin inhibit gastric acid secretion while soothing and healing ulcers and inflammation.

Chamomile Apigenin and other anti-inflammatories reduce swelling and help accelerate the healing of damaged tissues in the stomach and esophagus.

Calendula- Anti-inflammatory flavonoids speed up recovery from gastritis, ulcers, and reflux by stimulating tissue regeneration and cell repair processes.

For natural relief, steep 2 tablespoons each of marshmallow root, slippery elm, licorice root, chamomile flowers, and calendula petals in hot water for 10-15 minutes. Drink 3 times daily to coat, protect, and heal irritated digestive tissues.

Improving Gallbladder Function

Sluggish bile production can impair fat digestion and eliminate toxins leading to gallstone formation. Herbal cholagogues promote bile flow for improved gallbladder health.

Dandelion Root- Taraxacin increases bile output to aid digestion and elimination of wastes. This helps prevent gallstone formation.

Boldo Leaves- Alkaloids like boldine stimulate liver bile production and gallbladder contractions to boost bile flow through bile ducts.

Milk Thistle- Silymarin in milk thistle protects and repairs liver cells involved in bile synthesis and enhances bile solubility to prevent stones.

Peppermint- Menthol increases bile flow from both the liver and gallbladder while relaxing spasms to allow the passing of small stones.

Turmeric- Curcumin boosts the production and excretion of bile while decreasing inflammation allowing gallstones to pass more easily.

To improve gallbladder function combine 2 teaspoons each of dried dandelion root, boldo leaves, milk thistle seeds, peppermint leaves, and turmeric powder. Steep in hot water for 15 minutes before drinking daily.

Achieving Optimal Digestive Health with Herbal Teas

Maintaining a healthy, smoothly functioning digestive system is crucial for overall well-being. When digestion goes awry, it can negatively impact energy levels, nutrition, immunity, mood, and more. Herbal teas are a safe, effective way to both prevent and treat many common digestive disorders. The medicinal compounds found in botanicals can address underlying causes of gastrointestinal troubles ranging from inflammation to gut flora imbalances.

By incorporating gut-friendly herbal teas into your daily routine, you can gently cleanse, strengthen, and nourish your entire digestive tract.

Peppermint and Ginger Tea for General Belly Comfort

This classic herb combo contains volatile compounds that help relax the gastrointestinal tract, reduce inflammation, dispel gas, and stimulate digestion. The menthol in peppermint has a soothing, cooling effect on the intestines while easing spasms and pain. Gingerols in ginger suppress prostaglandins to reduce inflammation associated with poor digestion. Both herbs improve overall gastric motility and emptying.

To make a belly-comforting tea, add 1-2 teaspoons of freshly grated ginger root and a handful of fresh peppermint leaves to a tea infuser. Steep in 8 oz hot water for 5-10 minutes. The spicy-cool blend of ginger and mint will help settle the stomach while promoting healthy digestion. Drink after meals when experiencing abdominal discomfort, indigestion or sluggish digestion. This tea is also great for relieving nausea and motion sickness.

Fennel, Cumin, and Coriander Tea for Bloat Relief
This aromatic tea combination leverages the potent carminative properties of spices like fennel, cumin, and coriander to provide quick relief from bloating and gas pains. The volatile oils found in these herbs relax gastrointestinal muscles to help release trapped gas from the intestines. Fennel and coriander also improve bile flow and digestion to prevent future gas accumulation.

To whip up a fast bloat-busting tea, steep 1 tablespoon each of fennel seeds, cumin seeds, and coriander seeds in 6-8 oz hot water for 5-7 minutes. The distended belly usually starts deflating quickly once the warm, fragrant tea hits your stomach. Drink after meals to aid digestion and prevent post-meal gas and bloating. This tea also helps relieve colic pain in babies when the mother drinks it.

Licorice, Cinnamon, and Cardamom Tea for Acid Reflux
This soothing herbal tea combination can provide relief from the burning discomfort caused by acid reflux. Licorice root contains triterpenoids that help protect the esophageal lining from erosion by stomach acid. Cinnamon enhances gastric mucus secretions to create a barrier against reflux. And cardamom has natural antacid effects to neutralize excess acids.

To ease acid reflux discomfort, steep 1 tablespoon diced licorice root, 1 cinnamon stick, and 4 cardamom pods in 6-8 oz hot water for 10 minutes before straining and drinking 30 minutes after meals. This warming tea will coat your esophagus and help strengthen the lower esophageal sphincter to prevent painful acid backups. It's also delicious with a touch of raw honey.

Slippery Elm and Marshmallow Root Tea for Gastritis
The mucilaginous fibers found in demulcent herbs like slippery elm and marshmallow root make them ideal for coating and soothing inflamed tissues in the GI tract. When steeped, they become gelatinous and coat the mouth, esophagus, and stomach lining, providing relief from the burning pain of gastritis. They reduce inflammation and help protect against additional damage from stomach acid.

For a gut-coating digestive aid, simmer 2 tablespoons each of slippery elm bark powder and marshmallow root chunks for 10-15 minutes in 32 oz of water until thickened. Allow to cool and drink 1 cup 20 minutes before meals to coat and adhere to the stomach lining. This mucilaginous tea is excellent for healing gastritis, ulcers, and GERD naturally.

Dandelion Root and Milk Thistle Tea for Constipation
This herbal pairing works together to gently stimulate bile flow and intestinal contractions to relieve constipation while protecting and strengthening liver function. Bitter compounds in dandelion root increase bile output which in turn improves digestion and promotes regular bowel movements. Milk thistle guards liver cells while helping cleanse toxins for better bile production.

To get things moving, steep 1 tablespoon chopped dandelion root and 1 teaspoon milk thistle seeds in 6-8 oz hot water for 10 minutes. Drink once daily, ideally first thing in the morning on an empty stomach. This tea combination will help strengthen natural elimination patterns over time when drunk regularly. Be sure to also drink plenty of fluids.

Ginger, Peppermint, and Fennel Tea for Nausea

These three herbs are excellent natural remedies for quelling nausea, especially ginger. Ginger contains potent anti-emetic compounds called gingerols and shogaols that help calm nausea triggered by motion sickness, pregnancy, infections, medications, and more. Peppermint and fennel add additional stomach-soothing and gas-relieving actions.

For quick relief from nausea and vomiting, steep 2 tablespoons grated fresh ginger, 1 tablespoon dried peppermint leaves, and 1 teaspoon fennel seeds in 8 oz hot water for 10 minutes. Slowly sip the tea, allowing the aromatic liquid to coat your throat and settle your stomach. The first sign of relief usually comes within 5-10 minutes.

Chamomile, Lemon Balm, and Catnip Tea for Stress Relief
This relaxing tea blend works on soothing anxiety and tension that takes a toll on digestive health. Chamomile contains natural sedative compounds that induce calm and reduce stress hormone levels. Lemon balm elevates mood and eases stress while also improving digestion. And catnip relieves muscle spasms and tightness caused by chronic stress.

To promote relaxation and support healthy digestion, steep 2 tablespoons each of dried chamomile flowers, lemon balm, and catnip in 8 oz of hot water for 10 minutes. Sip this soothing tea 20-30 minutes before meals to dial down stress levels and allow proper digestion. The relaxing compounds help prevent stress-related indigestion.
Ginger and Turmeric Tea for Gallbladder Health

Ginger and turmeric make the perfect pairing for stimulating bile production and easing gallbladder discomfort. Gingerol boosts bile secretion to improve fat digestion while curcumin reduces gallbladder inflammation allowing for the easy passage of stones. Both compounds are potent antioxidants that protect liver cells.

For better gallbladder function, simmer 1 tablespoon freshly grated ginger and 1 teaspoon turmeric powder in 6-8 oz of water for 5-10 minutes. The bright, warm brew delivers powerful anti-inflammatory and bile-stimulating compounds with each sip. Drink daily to keep bile production regular and prevent gallstone formation.

Incorporating gut-friendly teas into your daily routine is an easy way to optimize every aspect of digestion. The medicinal compounds found in herbs and spices deliver healing benefits throughout the entire gastrointestinal tract – from mouth to colon. Drinking these teas regularly can help prevent many common digestive problems as well as relieve discomfort from issues like reflux, gas, nausea, constipation, and gallstones when they occur. Discover greater digestive wellness with the power of healing botanicals.

Restoring Digestive Wellness with Medicinal Teas

Achieving optimal digestive health is key to overall well-being, yet many people struggle with chronic issues like reflux, constipation, nausea, and bloating. Thankfully, certain herbs contain compounds that can help remedy digestive troubles in a safe, natural way without harsh side effects. Tannins tighten tissues, bitters stimulate secretions, volatile oils relax muscles, mucilaginous demulcents coat and soothe, and antimicrobials fight pathogens.

Incorporating medicinal herbal teas into your daily routine can provide effective, long-lasting relief from digestive woes while strengthening and protecting the entire GI tract. Discover some of the top research-backed botanicals for optimizing every aspect of your digestion.

Chamomile and Ginger Tea for Indigestion
This soothing combination helps settle the stomach while easing indigestion, gas, and bloating after meals. Chamomile contains natural anti-inflammatories like bisabolol that relax stomach muscles and reduce inflammation associated with indigestion. Ginger speeds up delayed gastric emptying which remedies that "heavy" discomfort. The gingerols also minimize gas production.

For relief after heavy meals, steep 2 tablespoons of dried chamomile flowers and 1 teaspoon of freshly grated ginger in hot water for 10 minutes. Drink slowly after eating. This aromatic tea will calm the stomach, reduce inflammation, and help digest problematic foods. The antispasmodic actions provide fast relief without drowsiness.

Peppermint, Fennel, and Ginger Tea for IBS
All three herbs in this tea contain compounds that target the most common IBS symptoms: pain, cramping, spasms, gas, and erratic motility. Peppermint and ginger relax intestinal smooth muscle to relieve spasms and improve mobility. Fennel eases bloating and gas production through its carminative effect.

To manage IBS flares, steep 2 tablespoons of dried peppermint leaves, 1 tablespoon of fennel seeds, and 1 teaspoon of grated ginger in 8 oz hot water for 10 minutes. Drink 30 minutes before meals to prevent painful post-meal GI spasms. This combo also reduces abdominal pain, bloating, and urgency when drunk after mealtimes.

Marshmallow Root and Slippery Elm Tea for Gastric Ulcers
The mucilaginous properties of demulcent herbs make them ideal for coating, soothing, and protecting irritated tissues in the GI tract. Marshmallow root and slippery elm contain polysaccharides that form a gel-like barrier against stomach acid and enzymes, allowing ulcers to heal.

To help heal ulcers, steep 3 tablespoons marshmallow root chunks and 2 tablespoons slippery elm bark powder in 32 oz hot water for 15 minutes until thickened. Allow to cool before drinking 1 cup 20 minutes before meals to coat and adhere to the stomach lining. The mucilage adheres firmly, shielding ulcers from further damage so they can heal.

Ginger, Turmeric, and Fennel Tea for Bile Reflux
This bright, aromatic tea blend can help settle bile reflux discomfort while also improving motility and bile production. Ginger and turmeric reduce inflammation in the stomach lining caused by acidic bile exposure. Fennel improves digestion and gut mobility to flush up bile before it refluxes.

For relief from the burning sensation of bile reflux, simmer 1 tablespoon ginger, 1 teaspoon turmeric and 1 tablespoon fennel seeds in 32 oz water for 10 minutes. Allow to cool and sip 30 minutes after meals. This healing combination will help strengthen your lower esophageal sphincter and stimulate bile flow to prevent painful bile backups.

Peppermint, Chamomile, and Lemon Balm Tea for Stress
This relaxing tea combo works to ease anxiety and tension that can negatively impact digestion. Peppermint and chamomile contain natural compounds that reduce stress signals to calm the nervous system. Lemon balm elevates mood and improves digestion.

Steep 2 tablespoons each of dried peppermint, chamomile flowers, and lemon balm in 8 oz hot water for 7-10 minutes. Drink 20-30 minutes before meals to lower cortisol levels and relax your digestive tract, allowing for better food breakdown and absorption. This tea also promotes restful sleep.

Slippery Elm and Marshmallow Root Tea for Diarrhea
The mucilaginous demulcents slippery elm and marshmallow root can provide soothing relief for inflammatory diarrhea like ulcerative colitis, Crohn's and IBS-D. When mixed with water, they become gelatinous and coat irritated intestinal tissues, easing inflammation and discomfort.

For relief from frequent loose stools, simmer 3 tablespoons slippery elm bark powder and 2 tablespoons of marshmallow root chunks in 32 oz water for 10-15 minutes until thickened. Allow to cool before drinking 1 cup on an empty stomach followed by small sips throughout the day. This will help firm up loose stools while healing inflamed intestinal tissues.

Dandelion, Burdock, and Chicory Tea for Liver Health
These bitter herbs help strengthen digestive function by stimulating bile flow, aiding digestion, and cleansing the liver. Dandelion and chicory increase bile output, which carries waste and toxins out of the body. Burdock root clears accumulated metabolites, uric acid, and heavy metals from the liver and bloodstream.

For improved liver health and digestion, steep 2 tablespoons each of dried dandelion root, burdock root, and chicory root in 32 oz hot water for 15 minutes. Drink 1 cup daily either first thing in the morning or before bed to support liver function and bile production. This tea cleanses the liver while protecting liver cells.

The diverse compounds found in medicinal botanicals can bring relief to nearly every type of digestive complaint. Tannins tighten tissues, bitters and carminatives stimulate digestion, mucilaginous demulcents coat and soothe, and anti-inflammatories like ginger reduce swelling and discomfort. Make gut-healthy herbal teas part of your daily routine for optimal digestive wellness.

Herbal Teas for Complete Digestive Wellness:

Achieving optimal digestive health is essential for overall well-being. Herbal teas provide a natural, time-tested way to prevent and relieve many common gastrointestinal disorders without harsh side effects. Certain botanicals contain an array of beneficial compounds that address underlying causes of digestive troubles.

Tannins tighten tissues, carminatives reduce gas, bitters stimulate secretions, volatile oils relax muscles, demulcents coat and soothe, and antimicrobials fight pathogens. Incorporating medicinal herbal teas into your daily routine can strengthen, tone, and protect your entire GI tract for complete digestive wellness.

Peppermint and Ginger Tea for Improved Digestion
This classic tea pairing works synergistically to optimize digestion in multiple ways. Peppermint contains menthol, a volatile compound that relaxes intestinal muscles to improve mobility and nutrient absorption. Ginger speeds up gastric emptying to prevent that sluggish, bloated feeling after eating.

To support healthy digestion, add 1 tablespoon freshly grated ginger and 2 tablespoons dried peppermint leaves to a tea infuser and steep in 8 oz just-boiled water for 7-10 minutes. Sip this aromatic brew

20-30 minutes before meals to prime your GI tract for optimal digestion and nutrient assimilation.

Fennel, Cumin, and Ginger Tea for Gas and Bloating
Bloating and excessive gas can make simple activities uncomfortable. This carminative tea blend provides quick relief by helping your body expel built-up intestinal gas. Fennel and cumin contain volatile compounds like anethole and thymol that relax smooth muscles and allow trapped gasses to pass. Ginger also minimizes gas production.

For fast relief from a distended, gassy belly, steep 1 tablespoon each of fennel seeds, cumin seeds, and grated ginger root in 8 oz recently boiled water for 7-10 minutes. Drink slowly after meals. The aromatic oils will permeate your digestive tract, easing muscle spasms and releasing excess flatulence.

Marshmallow Root and Slippery Elm Tea for Heartburn
The demulcent properties of marshmallow root and slippery elm make them ideal for coating, soothing, and protecting irritated tissues from excess stomach acid. When mixed with water, they create a gelatinous mucilage layer that adheres to the esophageal lining, shielding it from erosion.

For relief from reflux discomfort, simmer 3 tablespoons marshmallow root and 2 tablespoons slippery elm bark in 32 oz water for 10-15 minutes until thickened slightly. Allow to cool before drinking 1 cup 20-30 minutes after meals to coat and adhere to your esophagus and stomach. This mucilaginous brew will prevent painful acid reflux.

Ginger, Peppermint, and Chamomile Tea for Nausea
This herb and spice medley provides soothing relief for all types of nausea, especially morning sickness. Ginger contains potent

anti-emetic compounds called gingerols that ease nausea by relaxing the stomach and improving digestion. Peppermint and chamomile add antispasmodic actions to suppress nausea triggers.

Steep 2 tablespoons grated fresh ginger, 1 tablespoon dried peppermint leaves, and 2 tablespoons dried chamomile flowers in 8 oz hot water for 7-10 minutes. Slowly sip this fragrant tea when nausea strikes. The herbs will quickly calm your stomach upset and help settle your insides. Drink as needed.

Licorice Root and Marshmallow Root Tea for Ulcers
Licorice root contains triterpenoids that help protect the stomach lining from excess acid and stimulate mucus production. This allows ulcers to heal. The mucilaginous compounds in marshmallow roots adhere firmly to ulcerated tissues to shield them from further damage while also reducing inflammation.

To help heal ulcers naturally, simmer 3 tablespoons dried licorice root and 2 tablespoons marshmallow root chunks in 32 oz of water for 15 minutes until thickened slightly. Drink 1 cup of this gelatinous tea 20 minutes before meals to coat, protect and soothe your stomach lining, allowing ulcers to heal.

Dandelion, Milk Thistle, and Artichoke Tea for Digestive Detox
This trio makes an excellent herbal tea for improving digestion and performing a gentle liver cleanse. Dandelion stimulates bile flow to aid digestion and elimination of toxins. Milk thistle strengthens and protects liver cells. Artichoke leaf helps regenerate liver tissues and improves gallbladder function for better bile flow.

For a digestive system cleanse, steep 3 tablespoons dried dandelion root, 1 tablespoon milk thistle seeds, and 2 tablespoons artichoke leaf extract powder in 32 oz hot water for 15 minutes. Allow to cool and drink 1 cup daily either in the morning or before bed for healthier digestion and enhanced liver function.

Slippery Elm and Marshmallow Root Tea for IBD
The demulcent mucilage formed when marshmallow root and slippery elm bark are mixed with water makes them ideal for coating and soothing inflamed intestinal tissues in disorders like Crohn's and ulcerative colitis. This gelatinous blend adheres firmly to the GI lining, protecting and healing it.

Simmer 3 tablespoons marshmallow root chunks and 2 tablespoons slippery elm bark powder in 32 oz water for 10-15 minutes. Allow to cool and drink 1 cup on an empty stomach followed by small sips throughout the day to coat and soothe irritation. This mucilaginous tea is excellent for healing IBD flare-ups and symptoms like urgent diarrhea.

Incorporating gut-healthy herbal teas into your daily routine can optimize every aspect of digestion for complete GI wellness. The diverse medicinal compounds found in plants provide natural relief for issues like gas, heartburn, constipation, and nausea without side effects. Discover greater digestive vitality with the healing power of botanicals.

Chapter 5

Cold Crusher: Echinacea and Elderberry Tea

Feeding off colds, flu, and respiratory infections is one of the most popular uses of herbal tea. Among the most clinically researched and effective herbs for immune defense against viruses and bacteria are echinacea and elderberry. Combining these two antiviral and anti-inflammatory powerhouses into a medicinal blend makes for a delicious preventative health tea.

Echinacea is a purple coneflower native to North America revered for its ability to stimulate white blood cell production and activity to heighten immune response. Regularly sipping echinacea tea may help reduce cold and flu incidence and duration. Its aromatic flavor combines nicely with the rich, deep berry notes of elderberry. High in vitamin C and antioxidants, elderberry demonstrates strong antiviral effects against cold and flu viruses like influenza B. Together these herbs pack an immune-bolstering punch.

You can find both echinacea and elderberry herbs in health food stores and herbal medicine shops. Look for the dried flowers, leaves, and roots of the Echinacea purpurea or pallida species. Elderberry is sold in dried berry or powder form. For optimal freshness and potency, source organic or ethically wildcrafted herbs from reputable suppliers. Store in airtight containers away from heat, light, and moisture.

To brew a cup of this dynamic medicinal duo:

Boil filtered water and pour it into a large mug. Let cool slightly.
Add 1 teaspoon dried echinacea and 1 teaspoon dried elderberry.
Cover and steep for 5-7 minutes.
Strain into your favorite mug using a fine mesh sieve or tea strainer.
Stir in a teaspoon of raw honey if desired. The honey has added antimicrobial benefits.
Sip slowly and enjoy the complex earthy, tangy flavors.
Drink 1-2 cups daily during cold and flu season to prevent infection. At the very first signs of a viral illness - fatigue, scratchy throat, sniffles - begin drinking several cups per day to support your body's immune response. The herbs' compounds stimulate your system's natural defenses against the invading microbes. Both children and adults can use this tea safely.

Immunity Ignitor: Astragalus, Lemongrass, and Ginger Tea

Warding off seasonal illness requires fortifying your defenses year-round. Sipping immune-enhancing herbs daily strengthens your internal resistance and resilience against whatever pathogens come your way. Combining adaptogenic astragalus with the uplifting notes of lemongrass and spicy heat of ginger makes for an aromatic Immunity Ignitor tea that metaphorically puts pathogens on notice!

Astragalus has an illustrious history in Traditional Chinese Medicine as an adaptogenic herb that tonifies vital energy and bolsters immunity. With its mild sweet taste and affinity for strengthening the lungs and spleen, astragalus blends smoothly with the citrusy, grassy flavor of lemongrass. Known in Ayurveda to ward off colds and congestion, lemongrass makes this mix bright and refreshing. Ginger's signature warmth rounds it out for an immunity-stoking infusion guaranteed to get your defenses fired up.

You can find organic astragalus root, lemongrass stalks, and ginger root in most natural grocery stores or online herbal shops. Look for plump, fresh-looking astragalus slices and lemongrass. Ginger should feel firm with smooth skin. Store the herbs in airtight containers away from heat, light, and moisture. Make sure to frequently restock your immunity trio to harness their freshest potency.

To brew up your own Immunity Ignitor tea:

Bring 4 cups of filtered water to a boil. Reduce to a simmer.
Add 3 TBSP astragalus root slices.
Add 4 lemongrass stalks, smashed.
Simmer for 30 minutes, covered.
Remove from heat and add 2 TBSP grated ginger.
Steep covered 10 minutes more.
Strain tea through a sieve into mugs.
Sweeten with lemon and honey if desired.
Drink 1-2 cups daily, ideally first thing in the morning to prime your inner defenses for the day ahead. The tea's vibrant flavors and aromas will energize your spirit while the herbs' compounds activate your immune cells. Drink more frequently as needed when feeling under the weather or highly stressed. Now let's explore each featured ingredient's immune-enhancing qualities:

Astragalus is a staple herb in Traditional Chinese Medicine renowned as a versatile adaptogen that enhances vitality, endurance, digestion, heart health, and immunity. The root has a sweet, mild taste and is commonly blended into soups and teas to boost wellbeing. Modern research is unveiling Astragalus' numerous health benefits, validating its historical esteem. In Chinese medicine, astragalus is said to tonify the lung and spleen qi, essentially invigorating the organs responsible for circulating oxygen and nutrients. Astragalus contains specialized polysaccharides that have been found to stimulate white blood cell production and activity. These immune-modulating effects make astragalus tea a valuable preventative tonic.

Anti-Inflammatory Infusion: Turmeric, Cinnamon and Black Pepper

Inflammation can wreak havoc on the body and negatively impact overall health in numerous ways. An overactive immune system triggers widespread inflammation, leading to joint pain, digestive issues, headaches, skin problems and a host of other concerns. By taming inflammation naturally with anti-inflammatory foods and herbs, you can soothe these issues and help your body function optimally.

One simple and delicious way to fight inflammation is with a warm, soothing cup of Anti-Inflammatory Infusion tea. This powerful blend contains three incredible ingredients that have been used for centuries in traditional healing practices to reduce inflammation in the body: turmeric, cinnamon, and black pepper.

Turmeric is arguably one of the most potent anti-inflammatory spices on the planet. The active compound in turmeric, curcumin, has been widely studied for its ability to inhibit inflammatory pathways and enzymes in the body. Research has uncovered that curcumin is highly effective at reducing markers of inflammation and oxidation. Additionally, it has been shown to improve symptoms in a diversity of inflammatory conditions, including arthritis, digestive disorders, atherosclerosis, and many more.

The range of health benefits from turmeric does not stop there. The golden-hued spice has also demonstrated antimicrobial effects in battling unwanted pathogens. It has antioxidant capabilities to neutralize free radicals that damage cells. Curcumin has even shown potential in preventing cognitive decline and alleviating depression. The applications of powerful turmeric truly seem endless. It is no wonder that it has been called "the spice of life" in India, where it has been revered for thousands of years as a healing remedy.

Zesty Citrus Immune Boost: Orange Peel, Rose Hips and Hibiscus

With so many threats lurking at every turn, from seasonal bugs to more serious viruses, boosting immunity is a wise preventative health measure. While proper rest, nutrition, and hygiene form a strong first line of defense, certain foods and herbs can provide additional reinforcement. Sipping on a warm, aromatic cup of herbal tea is a soothing way to nourish your body's natural defenses.

Zesty Citrus Immune Boost tea combines three powerful ingredients that possess impressive immune-enhancing effects: orange peel, rose hips and hibiscus. This vitamin C-packed blend offers a tangy citrus burst in each sip that awakens the senses and invigorates the body's infection-fighting warriors.

Orange peel might seem like a humble leftover from juicing, but it harbors a wealth of hidden health treasures. Those tossed rinds are among the most nutritious parts of the orange, densely packed with protective compounds. Dried orange peel contains up to 60 times more vitamin C than the juice and pulp. It also provides potent phytochemicals like polyphenols, terpenes and flavonoids that optimize immune cell activity.

Research confirms the peel exhibits antibacterial, antiviral, antifungal, and anti-inflammatory properties. The citrus flavonoids it contains are particularly effective at inhibiting viral reproduction and growth. Hesperidin demonstrates strong antiviral effects against numerous pathogens, including influenza, adenovirus, and rotavirus. Other polyphenols show promise for preventing the replication of RNA viruses.

These multifaceted immune-enhancing effects make orange peel a wise addition during cold and flu season. All it takes is one tablespoon of dried peel per cup of boiling water for 10 minutes to extract these mighty compounds into a vibrant infusion. Adjust to taste if you prefer a stronger or weaker citrus intensity.

Joining forces with orange peel in this blend is the humble but powerful rose hip. The bright red berry-like fruits left behind after a rose blossom blooms contain phenomenal vitamin C content. In fact, rose hips boast one of the highest concentrations of this crucial immune-boosting nutrient found in any plant.

One single tablespoon of the dried poppy seed pods provides 120 mg of vitamin C. That's over 100% of the recommended daily value, making rose hips an antioxidant-packed punch. Vitamin C stimulates the production of lymphocytes, phagocytes, and other protective white blood cells to seek and destroy pathogens.

Rose hips also contain a diversity of carotenoids and bioflavonoids that reinforce immunity. Research confirms this wild fruit reduces inflammation, fights infection, and enhances overall immune response. It exhibits antibacterial effects against numerous gram-positive and gram-negative bacteria.

The flavonoids contained in rose hips even inhibit viruses from attaching to cells and replicating. Plus, compounds like gallic acid and ellagitannins provide antioxidant power to protect cells from damage. Harnessing rose hips' nourishing benefits is as simple as steeping 1-2 tablespoons of dried hips per cup of hot water for 10 minutes.

Rounding out this vibrant citrus blend is hibiscus, a stunning ruby-hued flower that imparts gorgeous color and zippy tart flavor. But the benefits of hibiscus go far beyond beautifying your tea. It is chock-full of protective polyphenols and potent vitamin C to amplify the immune response.

Antiviral Ammunition: Garlic, Onion, Sage, and Thyme

Viruses are sneaky shapeshifters, constantly mutating to bypass our immune defenses. Just when we conquer one strain, a new variant crops up to wreak havoc all over again. To avoid getting caught in this endless loop of infection and recovery, we need versatile weapons in our medicinal arsenal that can combat viruses' many permutations.

Enter Antiviral Ammunition - an infusion brimming with sulfur-rich herbs that help thwart those villains before they can let loose and multiply. Garlic, onion, sage, and thyme are the potent plants that comprise this viral vanquishing brew.

Garlic is the star of the show, well known for its legendary antimicrobial effects. When garlic is cut or crushed, it releases allicin, an organosulfur compound responsible for its pungent aroma and many of its protective benefits.

Studies show that allicin blocks certain enzyme pathways and inhibits protein synthesis in bacterial, fungal, and viral cells. This impedes their ability to replicate and spread infection. Some strains have even become resistant to pharmaceutical antibiotics but still succumb to garlic's might.

Along with allicin, garlic contains other sulfuric compounds like ajoene, diallyl trisulfide, and S-allyl cysteine. In vitro and animal studies demonstrate these sulfurous molecules interfere with viral and bacterial adhesion, enter cells, proliferate, and induce apoptosis.

Specific viruses shown to be susceptible to garlic's organic sulfur compounds include influenza, cytomegalovirus, rhinovirus, viral pneumonia, herpes simplex 1 and 2, viral meningitis, and enteroviruses.

Garlic possesses broad-spectrum antimicrobial action against Gram-negative and Gram-positive bacteria, yeasts, fungi, and parasites as well. Some studies show greater potency from aged garlic extract compared to freshly crushed cloves.

So be sure to add garlic to your antiviral regimen in both forms. Crush or mince at least one fresh clove per day as seasoning or tea. Meanwhile, take an odorless aged garlic supplement to provide strong sulfurous viral and bacterial fighters. If the aroma or texture of garlic is unpalatable, supplements are an easy way to get high concentrations of garlic's active compounds.

What about onions, nature's mellower cousin to pungent garlic? It turns out onions contain similar organosulfur compounds, though in lower amounts. The distinctive strong sulfur scent upon cutting comes from propanediol oxide, which decomposes to form healing sulfoxides.

Onions provide anti-inflammatory, antioxidant, and antimicrobial effects much like garlic. Studies confirm onion juice and extracts suppress bacteria like E. coli, Pseudomonas, Proteus, Staphylococcus aureus, Mycobacterium tuberculosis, and Klebsiella.

Research also demonstrates activity against fungi like Aspergillus and Fusarium. Viruses shown to be susceptible include influenza A and B, respiratory syncytial virus, parainfluenza, and potentially HIV.

Onions activate immune cells like macrophages that engulf and destroy pathogens. The organosulfur compounds inhibit microbial adherence, metabolism, and replication. Particularly potent against viruses is quercetin, an antioxidant flavonoid concentrated in onion peels.

Now that you understand the merits of each herb, let's dive into how to mix up a steaming hot cup of Antiviral Ammunition to defend against those villains aiming to sabotage your systems:

Antiviral Ammunition Tea
Serves 2

Ingredients:

3 garlic cloves, crushed or minced
¼ onion, chopped
1 tablespoon fresh sage leaves (or 2 tsp dried)
1 tablespoon fresh thyme leaves (or 2 tsp dried)

32 ounces boiling water
Lemon wedges and honey to serve
Instructions:

Crush or mince garlic cloves. Chop onion and herbs.
Place all ingredients in a saucepan or tea kettle.
Pour in boiling water and allow it to steep for at least 10 minutes.
Strain tea through a fine mesh sieve into mugs.
Squeeze lemon juice and drizzle honey to taste.
Ideally, sip this aromatic infusion fresh for maximum potency. But cooled leftover tea can be stored refrigerated in an airtight container for up to 3 days. The longer infusion time coaxes out those antimicrobial oils that combat unwanted pathogens.

Feel free to adjust the proportions of each ingredient to suit your tastes. Start with equal amounts of onion, sage, and thyme along with a trio of minced garlic cloves per serving. Then tweak the recipe over time to create your optimal balanced antiviral ammunition.

Certain ingredients may become more prominent at times when you need to target specific problematic pathogens. For example, amp up the garlic during flu season or increase onion and sage if dealing with a viral or fungal infection. Get to know each ingredient and how it works synergistically so you can customize the tea to meet your unique needs.

If the flavor of raw garlic and onion is too intense, consider roasting or sautéing them first to mellow the bite. You can also take garlic capsules separately from drinking the herbal tea. Supplementing with aged garlic extract is an easy way to get antimicrobial benefits without the pungent flavor.

However, you choose to incorporate these fabulous phytochemical-rich foods into your routine, making them a regular habit is key to enhancing resilience. Use Antiviral Ammunition as the foundation then build upon it with other immune-boosting herbs like ginger, elderberry, and reishi as desired.

Here are some recommended ways to work this protective infusion into your wellness regimen:

Make a large batch and drink daily during cold and flu season
Sip when traveling or around people who are sick
Gulp at first signs of illness to stop invasion in its tracks
Drink throughout the day at the onset of any suspected infection
Steam face over the aromatic tea to clear sinuses and treat respiratory illness topically
Use leftovers for cooking beans, soups, grains or roasted veggies
Combine with bone broth for an ultra-restorative and antiviral soup
However you put this virus-vanquishing blend to work, know that each warming sip provides an army of antimicrobial molecules. Let's take a closer look at some of the most prominent active compounds housed within these everyday aromatic herbs and spices:

Garlic:

Allicin - This organosulfur is released when garlic is cut/crushed. Powerful antiviral and antibiotic effects come from this compound.

Ajoene - This garlic extract component interferes with integrin-dependent processes in viruses and bacteria, preventing adhesion and spread.

S-allyl cysteine - Detoxifies harmful free radicals and exhibits anti-influenza activity.

Diallyl trisulfide - Garlic oil component activates immune T-cells and suppresses active viral infection.

Melanoidins - Formed during heat processing of garlic, these exhibit antiviral activity against influenza A.

Onion:

Quercetin - Abundant antioxidant flavonoid concentrated in skins that impede viral influenza activity, poliovirus, and others.

Propyl disulfides - Volatile sulfurous compound that inhibits viral enzymes necessary for replication.

Allium Cepa agglutinin - Hemagglutinin component that disrupts pathogens' cellular membrane integrity.

Luteolin - An antioxidant and anti-inflammatory flavonoid that inhibits viral activation/replication.

Catechol - Phenol produced when onions are chopped. Powerful antioxidants fight viruses.

Sage:

Rosmarinic acid - Prominent antiviral polyphenol shown to prevent viral entry, fusion, and replication.

Apigenin & Luteolin: Flavonoids that combat hepatitis C, enterovirus, influenza, and herpes simplex.

Carnosic acid - Abundant in sage, this polyphenol inhibits viral neuraminidase enzymes and replication.

Thyme:

Thymol & Carvacrol - Volatile antimicrobial terpene compounds that permeate the cell membrane of pathogens.

Linalool & Eucalyptol - More antiviral/antibacterial terpenoid volatile oil components of thyme.

Flavonoids - Antioxidants like apigenin, naringenin & eriocitrin combat inflammation/free radicals.

As you can see, while each herb has its own profile of protective compounds, together they become a dynamic force against viruses and bacteria. The blended activity of allicin, sulfurous organics, antioxidant flavonoids, and antimicrobial terpenes provide multi-angle protection against unwanted pathogenic invaders.

By consuming these herbs in tea form, you gain the most potent benefits from water-soluble compounds that easily extract into the infusion. Meanwhile, take garlic and onion powders along with sage and thyme-based seasonings regularly in recipes too. This covers both the water and fat-soluble compounds for full antimicrobial action.

The next time you are under the weather, brew up a steaming mug of this Antiviral Ammunition tea. Its dynamic combination of health-promoting phytochemicals helps strengthen your defenses against those merciless microbial villains aiming to sabotage your systems.

Sipping this aromatic brew at the first sign of illness can stop an infection in its tracks if you listen closely to your body's signals. We all know that telltale scratchy throat or drained fatigue indicates microbial mischief makers are looking for a stronghold.

Arm yourself with Antiviral Ammunition and you have a powerful assist against seasonal sickness! But this tea is also beneficial year-round for preventing opportunistic bugs looking for any chance to bind and infiltrate your defenses.

Viruses are spread through contact with people and environments. Some evidence indicates that certain species can even remain dormant in nervous system tissues, waiting for the right moment of weakness to attack. Yikes!

We must safeguard ourselves on all fronts with adequate rest, stress-reduction, and immune-optimizing foods and herbs. Avoiding heavily trafficked zones during peak illness seasons is wise as well.

But despite best efforts, those virulent viruses have a way of finding us anyway. With antimicrobial teas like this one at the ready, you can combat trouble rapidly at first signs. Catching invaders quickly before they multiply and spread infection throughout the body and to others is crucial.

By staying vigilant to subtle signals and listening intently to your body's messages, prompt action enables a rapid reversal. Subtle scratchy throat, nasal stuffiness, low energy, and body aches are all early clues to brew a cup and stop attackers in their tracks!

In our go-go-go society, we have been conditioned to ignore subtle symptoms and push through. But allowing yourself to rest and flooding your system with antiviral support aids swift resolution. Listen and respond promptly!

Viruses are simply looking to replicate. They have no malicious intent, just coded biological imperative. Avoid villainizing the germs! We gain nothing through fear. Simply employ compassionate wisdom as you take action.

Approach any brewing battle gently but decisively. Arm yourself with knowledge of nature's remedies that science confirms are safe and effective when used intelligently. Set intentions on a smooth resolution for all - including your temporary viral inhabitants.

Avoid panicking or overreacting in attempts to obliterate. Find the optimal middle path between ignoring and attacking. You need not declare war! Simply create an internal environment through hygiene, rest, and herbs that is cleanly and calmly inhospitable.

The microorganisms will move along in search of more receptive terrain. This allows you to neutralize and dissolve the attempted invasion and block transmission calmly with minimum collateral damage.

Harness the wisdom of traditional medicine without adopting an adversarial viewpoint. Work with the highly intelligent microbial world respectfully for the benefit and growth of all life. This mentality helps avoid the downstream issues that come from waging war internally.

There are always symbiotic solutions that promote peaceful co-existence rather than attempting to dominate and destroy. Remember that viruses and bacteria play important roles in digestion, immunity, gene regulation, metabolism, and more.

We need not seek to eradicate all microbes in fear. Allow supportive herbs to restore equilibrium gently so our microbiome flourishes in balance once again.

The intelligence of nature always guides us back to harmony if we quiet our reactionary impulses and listen closely. Keep these principles in mind as you utilize Antiviral Ammunition and other supportive teas and herbs for staying well.

If a virus does successfully latch on and infection ensues, do not admonish yourself. Illness is never a personal failure. It is simply part of being human. We all become vulnerable at times for many reasons - stress, grief, burnout, hardship, fatigue.

Often we need these forced slowdowns to right ourselves when we veer off course or drain our reserves. View convalescence as a sacred initiation into deeper self-knowledge rather than something to resent.

What is the wisdom in this unwanted yet vital turning inward? Our intuitive voice becomes clearer in stillness. We can examine where energetic leaks and weaknesses may have occurred that allowed illness to gain a foothold.

Without distracting habits and busyness, we gain insight into what requires realignment within ourselves and in our lives. Subtle imbalances we overlook in busier times become glaringly evident when we are forced into quietude.

From this reflective space, we can address any mindsets, emotions, relationships or patterns that enable dysfunction and deplete reserves. We emerge energized and armed with self-knowledge to walk a healthier path.

Every illness delivers an invaluable opportunity to turn within, listen deeply, shed outdated ways, excavate buried feelings, and invite in the new. What needs release or renewal? This is sacred terrain.

Here you have permission to rest, restore, and re-emerge even stronger than before. Do not waste this precious window of deep healing by judging yourself harshly or lamenting temporary discomfort.

Instead, inhale the teachings that each day of stillness offers. Every twinge and ache carries wisdom about where to focus recovery. Each moment of boredom or frustration points to emotional spaces for self-discovery. Fully accept what this chapter of renewal requires.

Chapter 6

Skin Smoothing Green Tea and Matcha Face Scrub

Want a natural, affordable at-home facial that leaves your skin looking fresh and glowing? Whip up an easy green tea and matcha face scrub right in your kitchen. Both green tea and matcha powder are packed with antioxidants and anti-inflammatory plant compounds that nourish skin. When combined with gentle exfoliating ingredients, this scrub deeply cleanses, softens, and rejuvenates dull complexions. Discover how ingredients probably already in your pantry can create a spa-worthy treatment for radiant skin.

As discussed in previous chapters, green tea and matcha are both derived from the Camellia sinensis plant. Green tea leaves are simply dried after harvest, while matcha consists of stone-ground young green tea leaves. This fine powder contains ultra-concentrated levels of green tea catechins and other antioxidants. Epigallocatechin gallate (EGCG) is the most abundant and potent catechin, having strong anti-inflammatory and free radical scavenging effects. Applying green tea and matcha topically allows these compounds to work their magic directly on the skin.

Research shows that EGCG inhibits enzymes that break down collagen and elastin, the structural proteins that keep skin firm and elastic. Matrix metalloproteinases (MMPs) are responsible for gradually degrading these proteins over time, leading to wrinkles, sagging, and loss of that "youthful bounce" in the skin. By interfering with MMPs, catechins preserve collagen and elastin to soften fine lines and improve skin texture. The antioxidants in green tea and matcha also protect against environmental damage from UV rays, pollution, and chemicals that generate cell-damaging free radicals. Who needs pricey firming creams when your pantry holds natural alternatives?

Whip up the scrub right before use by mixing:

1 teaspoon matcha powder
1 teaspoon loose-leaf green tea or 2 green tea bags
1 tablespoon raw honey
1 tablespoon plain yogurt or milk
The lactic acid in yogurt gently exfoliates dead skin cells, while the honey softens and nourishes. Use about 2 teaspoons of the scrub on damp skin, massaging in circular motions before rinsing clean. Splash your face with cool water afterward for an instant pick-me-up. Use 1-2 times per week for best results. This scrub leaves skin fresh, renewed, and smoothed. The antioxidants continue protecting your complexion long after rinsing off.

Consider adding other skin-healthy ingredients like rice flour, oatmeal, lemon juice, or essential oils to customize your green tea face scrub. This quick beauty recipe harnesses the proven benefits of matcha and green tea for healthy, luminous skin. Brewed tea bags can be composted after use to reduce waste. With some simple ingredients from your kitchen, treat yourself to a spa-like scrub that brings out your natural radiance.

Skin Smoothing Green Tea and Matcha Face Scrub

Want a natural, affordable at-home facial that leaves your skin looking fresh and glowing? Whip up an easy green tea and matcha face scrub right in your kitchen. Both green tea and matcha powder are packed with antioxidants and anti-inflammatory plant compounds that nourish skin. When combined with gentle exfoliating ingredients, this scrub deeply cleanses, softens, and rejuvenates dull complexions. Discover how ingredients probably already in your pantry can create a spa-worthy treatment for radiant skin.

As discussed in previous chapters, green tea and matcha are both derived from the Camellia sinensis plant. Green tea leaves are simply dried after harvest, while matcha consists of stone-ground young green tea leaves. This fine powder contains ultra-concentrated levels of green tea catechins and other antioxidants. Epigallocatechin gallate (EGCG) is the most abundant and potent catechin, having strong anti-inflammatory and free radical scavenging effects. Applying green tea and matcha topically allows these compounds to work their magic directly on the skin.

Research shows that EGCG inhibits enzymes that break down collagen and elastin, the structural proteins that keep skin firm and elastic. Matrix metalloproteinases (MMPs) are responsible for gradually degrading these proteins over time, leading to wrinkles, sagging, and loss of that "youthful bounce" in the skin. By interfering with MMPs, catechins preserve collagen and elastin to soften fine lines and improve skin texture. The antioxidants in green tea and matcha also protect against environmental damage from UV rays, pollution, and chemicals that generate cell-damaging free radicals. Who needs pricey firming creams when your pantry holds natural alternatives?

Whip up the scrub right before use by mixing:

1 teaspoon matcha powder
1 teaspoon loose-leaf green tea or 2 green tea bags
1 tablespoon raw honey
1 tablespoon plain yogurt or milk
The lactic acid in yogurt gently exfoliates dead skin cells, while the honey softens and nourishes. Use about 2 teaspoons of the scrub on damp skin, massaging in circular motions before rinsing clean. Splash your face with cool water afterward for an instant pick-me-up. Use 1-2 times per week for best results. This scrub leaves skin fresh, renewed, and smoothed. The antioxidants continue protecting your complexion long after rinsing off.

Consider adding other skin-healthy ingredients like rice flour, oatmeal, lemon juice, or essential oils to customize your green tea face scrub. This quick beauty recipe harnesses the proven benefits of matcha and green tea for healthy, luminous skin. Brewed tea bags can be composted after use to reduce waste. With some simple ingredients from your kitchen, treat yourself to a spa-like scrub that brings out your natural radiance.

Lavender and Chamomile Steamer for Facial Steam

Feel like your skin needs a reset? A relaxing facial steam opens pores, softens skin, and helps wash away impurities. Enjoy this soothing spa treatment at home using two of nature's most calming herbs - lavender and chamomile. The aromatic steam replenishes moisture, while the medicinal vapors reduce inflammation, redness, and irritation. Discover how easy it is to create a customized herbal steam facial using ingredients from your kitchen.

Facial steaming offers numerous benefits for all skin types. The warm humidity gently opens pores to dislodge dirt, oil, and dead skin buildup. Steaming improves circulation and hydrates skin by increasing blood flow to the face. Opening pores allows products like masks, serums, and moisturizers to penetrate better. It's an ideal way to prep skin for extraction facials or before special events when you want a luminous glow. The overall result is thoroughly cleansed, softened skin that absorbs moisture better.

Adding aromatherapeutic herbs enhances the relaxing and cleansing effects. Chamomile and lavender are perfect choices. Chamomile comes from the small daisy-like flowers of Matricaria recutita. It contains volatile oils, flavonoids, and antioxidants that reduce skin inflammation, irritation, and redness. Soothing chamomile is ideal for sensitive skin prone to reactivity. Lavender has long been prized in herbal medicine for its calming effects. The flowers yield a versatile oil used to heal wounds, burns, and skin disorders in addition to reducing anxiety and stress. Lavender also has antimicrobial properties to combat acne-causing bacteria. Together, chamomile and lavender make the ultimate stress-relieving steam.

To create your herbal facial steam:

Boil 2 cups of filtered water and remove it from heat.
Add 3-5 drops of lavender essential oil, 4 chamomile tea bags, and optional herbs.
Slowly pour into a large bowl.
Drape a towel over your head and carefully hover your face 8-10 inches above the water.
Steam face for 5-10 minutes, keeping eyes closed.
Try adding other beneficial herbs like rosemary, thyme, calendula, fennel, or lemon balm. Green tea, rose petals, or hibiscus make soothing additions as well. After steaming, splash your face with

cool water and apply a facial mask or moisturizer. Use the herbal steam two to three times per week when the skin needs an extra glow boost. The relaxing scent along with opened pores and increased circulation rejuvenates dull, congested complexions.

Treat yourself to the relaxing ritual of home facial steaming using healing herbs from your own kitchen. Let the aromatic vapors soothe your mind while the moist heat nourishes your skin. Use this all-natural therapy anytime your complexion feels lackluster. Coupled with a nutritious diet and healthy lifestyle habits, herbal steams enhance your natural beauty.Beyond the immediate effects, incorporating facial steaming into your regular skin care provides lasting benefits. The heat and moisture essentially "train" your pores to open up, allowing them to excrete oil and toxins better long term. Dilated pores minimize the likelihood of clogged pores and acne breakouts. The increased blood flow also boosts nutrient delivery to keep skin healthy and nourished. Facial steams hydrate and plump up the complexion, smoothing out fine lines and wrinkles. Regular use will leave your skin radiant, dewy, and glowing.

Don't have fresh or dried herbs on hand? No problem! You can create an effective facial steam with just hot water. Simply fill a large bowl with very hot - not boiling - water. Drape a towel over your head to trap the steam and lean over the bowl with your eyes closed. Be sure to keep your face at least 10 inches above the water to avoid scalding. Steam for 5-10 minutes until your skin looks flushed. The pure water vapor softens skin, unclogs pores, increases blood flow, and encourages cellular turnover. Just be careful not to splash hot water on your face.

Rose Petal and Hibiscus Skin Tonic Tea

Reveal your most vibrant, youthful complexion by nourishing skin with herbal ingredients teeming with antioxidants and anti-aging compounds. Steeping rose petals and hibiscus together make a wonderfully fragrant tonic to brighten, tighten, and protect your skin when consumed as a tea. Enjoy this floral elixir daily for noticeable improvements in your skin's texture, tone, and overall glow.

Roses have been prized since antiquity for their beautiful blooms and intoxicating fragrance. The petals also impart powerful skin and health benefits. Abundant polyphenols like anthocyanins, quercetin, catechins, and gallic acid give rose petals excellent antioxidant and anti-inflammatory activity. Rose essential oil contains additional volatile compounds with antimicrobial properties to combat acne-causing bacteria. Rose oil applied topically boosts skin cell regeneration and collagen production for smoother, firmer skin. Internally, rose petal tea enhances circulation while fighting free radical damage that ages skin.

Hibiscus flowers offer similar skin-enhancing effects in a tart, cranberry-like tea. Multiple species are used to make hibiscus tea, most commonly Hibiscus sabdariffa. The bright red sepals - the leafy cup below the flower - impart a tart, berry-like flavor and pigment. Hibiscus contains substantial vitamin C for collagen synthesis and flavonoids that inhibit elastin breakdown. Antioxidant anthocyanins give hibiscus strong free radical scavenging power against oxidative skin damage that manifests as wrinkles and hyperpigmentation. Drinking hibiscus tea regularly hydrates and nourishes the skin from the inside out.

Brew 4-5 rose buds with 2-3 hibiscus flowers or tea bags per cup of water for a refreshing vitamin-packed tonic. Steep 10-15 minutes to extract the flowers' beneficial compounds. Sweetening with a bit of honey balances the tart hibiscus flavor, or add lemon juice and a dash of cayenne for a zingy mock Cosmo! Sip this skin-nourishing tea daily. Topically, try chilled hibiscus tea as an antioxidant toner. For an intensive treatment, simmer rose buds and hibiscus flowers into a strong concentrate. Use once cooled as a face mask or hair rinse to combat dullness.

While oral skincare may seem counterintuitive, remember that healthy, radiant skin starts from within. What we ingest provides the building blocks and nourishment for great skin. By regularly consuming roses, hibiscus, and other herbs rich in bioactive compounds, their vitamins, antioxidants, minerals, and phytonutrients reach the skin through the bloodstream. Feed your skin vital nutrition with herbs that enhance circulation, promote cell turnover, stimulate collagen, and thwart free radical damage for flawless, youthful skin. Treat yourself to this fragrant rose and hibiscus beauty tea daily.

Mint and Green Tea Refreshing Foot Soak

After a long day on your feet, treat your hard-working soles to a relaxing herbal foot soak. Steeping mint and green tea together make an invigorating foot bath that energizes tired feet, fights odor and softens rough skin. As an added bonus, just breathing in the refreshing herbal steam provides aromatherapeutic effects to melt away stress. Keep reading to learn how you can create this spa-like soak at home using simple ingredients.

Start by brewing a large pot of strong green tea. Japanese sencha or bancha green teas make excellent choices, but any high-quality green tea will do. Steep 2 tablespoons of loose-leaf tea or 2-3 bags in about 4 cups of just-boiled water for 5 minutes. This produces a concentrated tea to dilute in your foot bath. You can also use the leftover tea bags from your morning cup! Green tea's antioxidant polyphenols like EGCG constrict blood vessels to help tighten and tone skin. The small amounts of caffeine in green tea also energize and revive tired feet.

Next, add several handfuls of fresh mint leaves to the hot tea, or about ¼ cup of dried mint. Japanese peppermint, spearmint, or regular culinary mint all provide a soothing minty flavor. Crush the leaves before steeping to release more aromatic oils. Mint contains menthol, which provides a cooling, analgesic effect on sore feet and muscles. It also has natural antibacterial properties to combat foot odor caused by bacteria and fungi. Other optional detoxifying herbs to add include dried rosemary, thyme, sage, and calendula flowers.

Pour the hot tea into a large basin, bucket, or other foot bath container. Top off with enough hot water to cover ankles when soaking feet. The ideal temperature for comfortable soaking is about 100-110°F – hot enough to feel relaxing but not scalding. Add a few drops of stimulating essential oils like peppermint, rosemary, or eucalyptus if desired. Soak your feet for 15-20 minutes while breathing in the refreshing herbal aromas. Rinse feet with cool water when done to close pores. Follow with a moisturizing foot cream or oil massage.

The rejuvenating mint and green tea foot soak provides relaxation along with tangible skin and foot care benefits. The hot water opens pores to deep clean sweat, odor, and dead skin buildup. Softened skin means it's easier to scrub away calluses and rough spots. The antioxidants and mint provide anti-aging and antibacterial protection. Regular foot soaking improves circulation in feet and ankles to reduce swelling. It also simply feels divine after extended standing or walking. Keep a stash of green tea bags and dried mint on hand for whenever your feet need some TLC.

Turn your home into a DIY spa with the phenomenal perks of hot herbal foot soaking. The ritual allows you to unwind as the aromatic steam envelops your senses. Close your eyes, breathe deeply, and let tension melt away while nourishing skin, fighting odor, and reviving tired feet. Light some candles, put on relaxing music, and take this time to intentionally care for yourself. A cup of tea afterward is an extra bonus. With some simple ingredients from your kitchen, treat your hardworking feet to the royal treatment they deserve.

Beyond the immediate beautifying effects, giving your feet and ankles some regular TLC provides lasting health benefits as well. The hot water and botanical compounds help strengthen connective tissue and improve circulation over time. You'll notice improved skin texture and suppleness in your feet from the topical antioxidants. The heat speeds metabolism and toxin removal in feet and legs to prevent varicose veins. Overall, you achieve better stamina and reduced foot pain with routine soothing foot soaks.

Consider using your foot soak as an opportunity to apply a nourishing foot mask as well. Applying foot masks and exfoliants after soaking maximizes their absorption and effectiveness once pores are opened and dead skin is softened. Some easy DIY options include

Honey + lemon juice: Apply a mixture of raw honey and fresh lemon juice to freshly soaked feet. Leave on for 10-15 minutes before rinsing. Softens and deodorizes.
Sea salt scrub: Mix coarse sea salt with a bit of olive or almond oil and gently scrub soaked feet. Rinse and moisturize well afterward.
Avocado mask: Mash up half an avocado and apply on clean wet feet. Soak your feet for 10-15 minutes before rinsing. Richly moisturized.

Oatmeal scrub: Grind ½ cup oats into a powder and mix with warm water or milk to form a paste. Gently scrub feet and rinse. Soothes irritation.

Remember to thoroughly dry your feet and apply foot cream or oil after using any masks or scrubs. Take this time to massage feet as well to boost circulation and provide therapeutic stress relief.

Clarifying Chrysanthemum and Burdock Root Rinse

For hair that's healthy, strong, and impossibly shiny, try incorporating herbal hair rinses into your beauty routine. Making infused herbal tea with chrysanthemum and burdock root creates a clarifying rinse that removes buildup, prevents dandruff, and stimulates hair follicles for faster growth. The simple practice of pouring this tea blend over hair after shampooing provides noticeable benefits for nourished, dandruff-free locks with each use.Chrysanthemum tea is wildly popular in China and is made from the dried flowers of the chrysanthemum plant. It has a delicate floral aroma and refreshing vegetal taste. Beyond drinking as a tea, chrysanthemum has a long history of use in hair tonics and scalp treatments. Compounds like flavonoids, saponins, linoleic acid, and polysaccharides give chrysanthemum anti-inflammatory, anti-microbial, and follicle-stimulating effects. Rinsing hair with chrysanthemum tea helps eliminate dandruff, itchy scalp, and inflammation for healthier growth.

Pairing chrysanthemum flowers with burdock root provides additional scalp-purifying benefits. The deep roots of the Arctium lappa burdock plant are renowned in herbal medicine for removing toxins and residues. Inulin fiber and powerful plant compounds clear away the buildup, dirt, and oil at the roots. Rinsing with burdock eliminates impurities weighing down hair at the scalp for improved volume. The antioxidants also combat free radical damage from styling products, chemical treatments, and pollutants that can degrade hair over time.

Brew a large batch of this dynamic tea by steeping 2 tablespoons each of dried chrysanthemum flowers and burdock root per 4 cups of hot water for at least 10 minutes. Allow to fully cool before using - hot tea can damage hair. After shampooing, slowly pour the cooled tea over your hair from roots to ends. Massage into the scalp and let sit for 5-10 minutes before rinsing out. Shampooing washes away the tea's beneficial compounds, so use it as a final rinse instead. Repeat 1-2 times per week for best results. Comb through some leave-in conditioner post-rinse to keep ends hydrated.

Use this soothing chrysanthemum burdock rinse anytime your hair needs a deep clean. The gentle botanicals remove residue buildup without stripping locks. Benefits include cleansed, dandruff-free scalp, purified hair follicles for healthy growth, more volume by eliminating weighed-down roots, preserved moisture and shine, reduced hair loss from improved scalp health, and protection against free radical and UV damage.

Beyond the immediate beautifying effects, regular use strengthens hair to prevent damage long-term. The plant nutrients nourish follicles for optimal growth cycles resulting in faster growth over time. Hair becomes more resistant to breakage thanks to antioxidants neutralize free radicals from styling and environmental factors. Scalp buildup can stunt follicles, so keeping roots cleanly purged preserves growth.

Treat your scalp and strands to these botanical benefits with a relaxing cup of aromatic chrysanthemum burdock tea. While the herbs seep, drink the rest, as the compounds that beautify hair impart internal health benefits as well. The simple ritual of a post-wash herbal hair tea rinse naturally enhances shine, growth, and overall scalp and hair wellness.

Beyond chrysanthemum and burdock, experiment with other hair-healthy herbs in your rinses. Adapt the basic recipe using ingredients you likely already have on hand. Use black tea for deeper cleansing since the tannins remove oil and residue. Try chamomile, rosemary, and mint for their scalp soothing properties to combat dandruff. Hibiscus, amla, and marigold provide vitamin C to boost collagen and circulation. Horsetail, nettle, and oat straw add strength, reduce shedding, and mend split ends. Green tea, cloves, and sage preserve color by preventing UV and free radical damage. Rose petals, lime, and calendula enhance shine and add silky texture.

You can use pre-made herbal tea bags for convenience or buy herbs in bulk to create your own signature blends. Mix and match based on your hair needs like clarifying, volumizing, damage repair, etc. Specific hair issues like oily roots, dry ends, and color-treated hair benefit from targeted botanical rinses. Infuse into different oils like coconut or olive oil for deeper penetration. Tea tree and lavender essential oils also provide antimicrobial and soothing properties.

Anti-Aging Cinnamon, Rhodiola, and Goji Berry Tea

Feel yourself looking a bit dull and weary lately? The constant stresses and environmental assaults of modern life can visibly age us prematurely. Fortunately, nature provides a wealth of anti-aging compounds to help restore a glowing, youthful complexion. Sipping an herbal tea with cinnamon, rhodiola, and goji berries daily delivers a powerhouse of antioxidants, vitamins, and nutrients for skin rejuvenation from within. Discover how these herbs work together to smooth fine lines, improve elasticity, and reveal your most radiant skin at any age.

Cinnamon is one of the most aromatic and delicious spices used in cooking and baking. But cinnamon also has an impressive roster of health and anti-aging benefits. The bark contains antioxidant polyphenols called procyanidins that enhance skin cell regeneration and collagen synthesis. This helps reduce wrinkles and maintain youthful elasticity. Cinnamon also improves circulation to nourish skin and provide a healthy glow. Its anti-inflammatory properties calm redness and irritation as well. Just a half teaspoon amps up the antioxidant content of any herbal tea blend.

Rhodiola rosea is an adaptogenic herb popular for reducing the damaging effects of stress. Sometimes called "golden root" or "rose root," Rhodiola helps the body adapt to all kinds of stresses. In the skin, the active compounds rosavin and salidroside scavenge free radicals caused by UV rays, poor diet, lack of sleep, and environmental pollutants. Minimizing this oxidative damage prevents premature aging. Rhodiola also promotes circulation, hydration, and skin cell renewal. The calming adaptogenic actions also curb wrinkle-causing facial expressions!

Adding antioxidant-packed goji berries takes this tea's anti-aging powers up another notch. These tiny red berries contain over 20 vitamins and minerals, amino acids, and high amounts of zeaxanthin - an antioxidant that filters out UV rays. Goji polyphenols increase hyaluronic acid in skin for improved moisture retention and suppleness. The berries also reduce collagen degradation and stimulate immune cells that remove waste from skin cells. This improves tone, elasticity, and brightness.

Brew 2 tsp each dried cinnamon bark, chopped rhodiola root, and whole goji berries with 4 cups of hot water for 10 minutes. Strain, let cool, and drink daily. The cinnamon lends warmth, rhodiola provides an earthy taste, and goji berries impart a raisin-like sweetness. The consistency can be tweaked by adjusting the steeping times and ratio of each herb. Enjoy this rejuvenating tea daily for smoother, firmer, more luminous skin that defies your age.

Anti-Aging Cinnamon, Rhodiola, and Goji Berry Tea

While the compounds in this tea work from the inside out to restore skin at the cellular level, consider also using topically for added benefits:

Make a face spray using strongly brewed cooled tea. Spritz skin after cleansing for an antioxidant boost.
Mix the cooled tea with plain yogurt or mashed avocado for a deeply nourishing face mask.
Combine with coconut or olive oil and massage directly onto the skin for an intensive moisturizing treatment.
Soak a soft cloth in the tea and use it as a warm compress to relax facial muscles and open pores before applying products.
Add the leftover herbs to your bath as a rejuvenating soak for your entire body.
With daily ingestion and direct skin application, you get the maximum anti-aging and protective advantages from these herbs. Be patient and consistent, as it may take a few weeks to notice major improvements in your skin's texture, tone, and vibrancy. But soon you'll be hooked on this Ayurvedic elixir for eternal youth!

The cinnamon, Rhodiola, and goji berry combo makes a delicious triple threat to combat skin aging on all fronts: collagen breakdown, oxidative stress, moisture loss, UV damage, inflammation, decreased circulation, and slowed cell turnover. Savoring a cup daily feels indulgent, while the herbs work their magic on your complexion.

While this blend shines for maturing skin, it provides anti-aging and protective advantages for all complexions:

Teens: Sugary, fried, and processed foods combined with lack of sleep often show the first signs of damage and accelerated aging in teens. The heavy antioxidant content of this tea combats inflammation and free radical formation for a clear, even-toned complexion free of redness and breakouts.

20s: Estrogen levels start declining in the 20s leading to moisture loss. This tea's circulation and hydration benefits keep skin supple and prevent early-onset fine lines. The adaptogenic and collagen-protective actions also minimize signs of stress.

30s: Collagen production slows down in the 30s causing the first visible wrinkles. The procyanidins and vitamins here stimulate new collagen and keep it strong to delay wrinkling and sagging.

40s: Menopause and weathering from sun exposure accelerate aging in the 40s. This tea's antioxidants provide defense from further environmental damage. The herbs replenish moisture and improve elasticity.

50s and beyond: Mature skin gets thinner, drier, and more prone to wrinkling without sufficient collagen. This tea's anti-inflammatory, and antioxidant nutrients maintain youthful thickness and hydration while increasing plumpness.

Chapter 7

Kidney Cleanser - Dandelion, Nettle and Cranberry Tea

The kidneys play a vital role in eliminating toxins and waste from the body through urine production. However, the consistent accumulation of toxins from environmental pollutants, medications, and poor diet can overwhelm the kidneys over time. This chapter will explore creating an herbal kidney cleanse tea with dandelion, nettle, and cranberry to support the kidneys' natural detoxification processes.

Dandelion is an unassuming weed that grows prolifically in lawns and meadows worldwide. However, this plant is so much more than a nuisance to gardeners. Dandelion has been used for centuries in traditional healing systems for its cleansing, diuretic, and nutritive properties. The leaves, roots, and flowers are all used medicinally. Dandelion leaf is a natural diuretic that increases urine output to flush the kidneys. The root contains inulin, a prebiotic fiber that supports healthy gut flora linked to reduced kidney inflammation. Dandelion is also high in potassium, slowing potassium loss in the urine caused by some diuretics. The flowers are packed with antioxidant flavonoids that reduce inflammation and cell damage.

For the kidney cleanse tea, the dandelion leaf is the ideal part of the plant to use. Add 2 teaspoons of dried dandelion leaf per cup of hot water and steep for 5-10 minutes. This simple tea taps into dandelion's diuretic effects to increase urine production and filtration through the kidneys. Be sure to drink plenty of extra fluids when using dandelion-leaf tea to stay hydrated. Those with digestion issues may notice some stomach upset from dandelion's bitterness, so adding lemon, ginger or honey can improve the flavor.

Nettle leaf compliments dandelion leaf perfectly in a kidney cleansing tea. Stinging nettle gets its common name from the tiny irritating hairs covering the leaves and stems that release histamine, acetylcholine, and other chemicals when touched. Once stinging nettles are dried or cooked, the stinging chemicals are neutralized. Nettle leaf is another stellar herb for supporting kidney health and function. It works similarly to dandelion as a diuretic while also reducing inflammation in the kidneys and urinary tract. Research suggests nettle blocks inflammatory pathways involving NF-kB and COX enzymes. For the tea, add 1 teaspoon of dried nettle leaf along with the dandelion leaf for a double-diuretic kidney cleansing effect.

The third ingredient in this powerful kidney cleanser tea is dried cranberry fruit. Cranberries contain phytochemicals like proanthocyanidins that prevent bacteria like E. coli from adhering to the lining of the bladder and urinary tract. This makes cranberry an effective remedy for urinary tract infections. Cranberry's anti-adhesion benefits also extend to the kidneys, helping flush out any invasive bacteria. Add 1 teaspoon of dried cranberry fruit to the dandelion leaf and nettle leaf tea concoction for the full kidney cleansing infusion. Drink 1-2 cups of this tea daily for 1-2 weeks to flush the kidneys. Those with kidney disease should consult their doctor before using diuretic herbs like dandelion and nettle leaf. Otherwise, this tea is safe for most people.

The beauty of this kidney cleanse tea is that all the ingredients can easily be foraged or grown in the garden. Dandelions and nettle grow wild in many parts of the world. Just be absolutely certain you have properly identified dandelion and stinging nettle before harvesting. Forage dandelion leaves from yards that haven't been treated with herbicides or other chemicals. Harvest nettle leaves using thick gloves before the plant flowers when histamine levels peak. Choose young leaves for both herbs. Cranberries can be found fresh in autumn and dried year-round. Turn to reputable herb suppliers for the highest quality pre-dried herbs if foraging isn't possible.

As potent diuretics, dandelion, and nettle leaf encourage frequent urination, which is helpful for flushing the kidneys but could be inconvenient at work or school. The tea is best consumed at home in the evening before bed. Be sure to drink at least 8 cups of water throughout the day while using this tea to avoid dehydration. Don't overdo the dandelion and nettle by steeping longer than recommended since this can irritate the stomach and kidneys. Taking occasional breaks from the tea for a few days is wise as well. Listen to your body's response and adjust your usage accordingly.

Beyond the symptomatic relief of increased urination, this herbal tea supports kidney health on a cellular level. The antioxidants in dandelion, nettle, and cranberry reduce free radical damage to kidney cells and tissues. They also fight systemic inflammation that can impact kidney function. Drinking kidney cleanse tea for 1-2 weeks as part of a seasonal detoxification regimen gives your kidneys an herbal boost and helps optimize their performance long-term. By combining time-tested natural herbs, you can take control of your kidney health and experience the benefits of improved detoxification.

Liver Detox - Milk Thistle, Burdock, and Red Clover Tea

The liver is the body's primary filtration system, working tirelessly to metabolize nutrients, drugs, hormones, and environmental toxins. With chronic exposure to substances like alcohol, medications, pesticides, and pollutants, the liver often becomes congested and sluggish. Luckily, certain healing herbs have an affinity for the liver and can stimulate cleansing detoxification. A simple tea blending milk thistle, burdock root, and red clover make the perfect daily liver tonic. These herbs complement each other to protect liver cells, increase bile flow, and enhance the elimination of waste.

Milk thistle is regarded as the premier herb for liver health and regeneration. The active compounds in milk thistle are a group of antioxidant flavonoids collectively called silymarin. Milk thistle extracts standardized to 70-80% silymarin are commonly used therapeutically for liver disease. However, milk thistle tea utilizing whole ground seeds also confers benefits. The seeds are rich in protein, essential fatty acids, and key minerals like phosphorus, zinc, and selenium that support normal liver function. Milk thistle strengthens liver cell membranes, blocking the entrance of toxins and waste products. As a powerful antioxidant, it also helps halt free radical damage to liver cells caused by alcohol, medications, pollution, and the byproducts of metabolism.

For the liver detox tea, use 1-2 teaspoons of crushed milk thistle seeds per cup of freshly boiled water. Allow the tea to steeply cover for 20 minutes to fully extract the seeds' nutritional compounds. The tea will turn a brownish-red color and develop a mild, earthy taste. You can enhance the flavor by adding a teaspoon of raw honey. Drink 1-2 cups of milk thistle tea daily for liver cleansing effects.

Milk thistle is very safe and can be used long-term, although taking occasional breaks is wise. Some people report looser stools from the increase in bile flow. Reduce the milk thistle amount or discontinue use if this becomes uncomfortable.

The third liver-loving herb that rounds out this herbal tea is red clover. Red clover is a staple in traditional medicine across Asia, Europe, and North America, used topically for skin ailments and internally as a cleanser. Red clover contains a spectrum of essential nutrients like thiamine, niacin, vitamin C, calcium, chromium, and magnesium. It is rich in anti-inflammatory isoflavone phytoestrogens that both protect the liver and enhance detoxification. Research confirms red clover's antioxidant, bile-stimulating, and tissue-regenerating effects in animal liver injury models. For the tea, add 1 teaspoon of dried red clover blossoms per cup of hot water for a hint of sweetness to balance the burdock's bitterness. Allow the tea to steep for at least 10 minutes before drinking 1-2 cups daily.

You can purchase dried milk thistle, burdock root, and red clover from most health food stores and online herb retailers. However, growing your own herbs guarantees freshness and potency. Milk thistle grows readily from seed, thriving in a sunny, dry spot in the garden. Harvest the seed pods in summer when they turn brown. Burdock root can be planted in spring from seed, then dug up in autumn when the roots are large and the inulin content peaks. Hang plants upside down to dry before collecting the seeds and roots. Red clover also grows easily from seed in fields and garden beds. Gather the pinkish-purple flower heads during summer when in bloom. Place herbs on screens or hang bundles to air dry out of sunlight before storing for tea.

Resetting your liver function is one of the best things you can do for whole-body health and detoxification. Your liver filters over a quart of blood every minute to remove toxins and produce vital proteins, hormones, and cholesterol. When overworked and congested, the liver cannot perform optimally. Simple herbs like milk thistle, burdock, and red clover have been used medicinally for centuries to cleanse and care for the liver. By incorporating this nourishing tea into your routine, especially after periods of rich eating, drinking, or stress, you can refresh your liver for improved long-term wellness.

Lymph Mover - Red Clover, Cleavers & Calendula Tea

The lymphatic system is an intricate network of tissues and organs that transport lymph fluid, a clear liquid containing white blood cells and waste products. This waste-removal system complements the circulatory system to keep the body's tissues nourished and detoxified. However, sedentary lifestyles, chronic stress, food sensitivities, and toxic overload can congest the lymph, leading to inflammation and illness. Herbs such as red clover, cleavers, and calendula make up a gentle, effective lymph-moving tea to stimulate circulation and drainage in the lymphatics.

The primary herb in this formula is red clover, a wild flowering plant common in meadows and roadsides. Red clover has an expansive tradition of use as an herbal cleanser, expectorant, skin healer and bitter tonic. Studies confirm red clover contains phytoestrogenic isoflavones, salicylate anti-inflammatories, antioxidants, and vitamins that enhance immune function and fluid flow. Red clover specifically targets lymph circulation. The isoflavones biochanin A and formononetin in red clover help thin and drain congested lymph fluid so waste can be filtered from tissues.

To make the lymph moving tea, add 2 teaspoons of dried red clover blossoms per cup of hot water. Steep the tea covered for at least 10 minutes to fully release the red clover's medicinal components. Red clover imparts a mildly sweet, flowery flavor to the infusion. You can enhance the taste by adding lemon juice, ginger, or raw honey. Drink 1-3 cups daily. Red clover is very gentle and suitable for daily use for periods of time up to one month. Allow a week break before resuming if needed. Those taking pharmaceutical estrogen medications should consult their doctor before using red clover.

Blood Purifier - Burdock, Yellow Dock & Neem Tea

The blood is the river of life, delivering oxygen and nutrients while ushering away metabolic waste products. When this purification system is overloaded with toxins, the result is systemic inflammation and impaired tissue function. Herbs that "purify" the blood assist the body's organs detoxification in filtering out inflammatory wastes and restoring optimal circulation. Three herbs renowned for their blood-cleansing abilities are burdock root, yellow dock root, and neem leaf. Combined in tea, they provide a powerhouse blend to rejuvenate the blood.

Burdock is the premier blood purifier in this formula. A member of the daisy family, this common weed has large tap roots filled with medicinal benefits. Burdock root contains unique lignans, quercetin, and other polyphenols that balance hormone levels, reduce inflammation, and protect liver cell health. The inulin fiber in burdock also soothes gut inflammation that underlies many systemic issues. With regular use, burdock root improves the flow of bile and urine to filter toxic residues from the blood. Science validates burdock's ability to protect against liver cell mutation and damage from toxic chemicals and heavy metals.

For the blood-purifying tea, use 1-2 teaspoons of dried burdock root per cup of water. Burdock root should be decocted, or gently simmered for 20-30 minutes, to extract maximum benefits. The resulting tea has an earthy, bitter taste due to burdock's unique medicinal components. Adding lemon, ginger, licorice root or honey mellows the flavor. Drink 1-2 cups daily, ideally 30 minutes before meals to enhance nutrient absorption. Burdock root is very safe when taken regularly, although some people notice looser stools or more frequent night urination from the diuretic effects.

The second herb in this formula, yellow dock root, has overlapping benefits with burdock as a premier "blood cleanser." Yellow dock belongs to the buckwheat family and thrives in wetlands and disturbed soils. The long taproot grows 8-12 inches in length and contains concentrated phytochemicals that stimulate detoxification in the liver, kidneys, and colon. These include anthraquinones, which support regular bowel movements, and tannins and iron, which build healthy blood. Yellow dock specifically improves the function of the spleen to filter old red blood cells and recycle iron.
Heavy Metal Detox Tea - Cilantro, Chlorella & Orange Peel

Environmental heavy metal toxicity is an escalating health threat in modern times. Heavy metals such as lead, arsenic, cadmium, mercury, and aluminum are ubiquitous in the atmosphere, soil, and water supply due to pollution and contamination. When these metallic compounds accumulate in the body faster than they can be eliminated, oxidative damage and inflammation result. Herbs such as cilantro, chlorella, and orange peel work synergistically to bind and escort heavy metals out of the body safely. Brewed together as a tea, they provide a gentle daily heavy metal detoxification aid.

Cilantro, also known as coriander leaf, is the superstar ingredient in this formula, with extensive research validating its ability to chelate and eliminate heavy metals through urine excretion. Cilantro's leaves and stems contain chlorophyll, flavonoids, polyphenols, and specific chelating compounds that bind to metal ions. This prevents their absorption and tissue accumulation while enhancing their secretion into bile and urine. Studies confirm cilantro significantly increases urinary excretion of lead, aluminum, tin, and mercury in animal subjects. The lead-chelating effect also holds true in humans based on emerging clinical research.

To make the tea, add a handful of fresh cilantro leaves and stems to 4-5 cups of hot water and steep for 15 minutes. The resulting tea has a refreshing, citrusy, green flavor. For convenience, substitute 2-3 teaspoons of dried cilantro leaf per cup of water and steep 10 minutes. Drink 2-4 cups of cilantro tea daily for 2-4 weeks to flush heavy metals. Cilantro is very safe and can be consumed regularly in food and tea. Those taking pharmaceutical medications should check for potential interactions with cilantro's unique detoxifying actions.

Chlorella, a blue-green algae, provides the perfect partner to cilantro in this tea. Rich in antioxidants like carotenoids and chlorophyll, chlorella binds tightly to heavy metals to prevent intestinal absorption and increase elimination. The tough cell walls of chlorella retain their structural integrity through digestion, allowing the algae cells to trap heavy metals and escort them out. Clinical research confirms chlorella reduces methylmercury absorption, increases its distribution to tissue for drainage, and enhances its urinary excretion. Lead, cadmium, and aluminum binding have also been demonstrated.

For the tea, add 1 teaspoon powdered chlorella to the hot cilantro tea and stir well to disperse. You can gradually increase the chlorella amount over time up to 1 tablespoon per cup as your body acclimates. Chlorella adds a noticeably green color and slightly grassy flavor to the tea which many people find appealing. Drink 2-4 cups per day. Chlorella does have a detoxifying effect of "mobilizing" metals stored in the body for elimination so mild symptoms like headaches or fatigue can sometimes occur when first using it. Starting slowly helps minimize this.

Orange peel makes the perfect final addition to pull heavy metals from tissue storage sites so they can be bound to cilantro and chlorella for excretion. The citrus peel contains antioxidant limonoids like d-limonene that protect the liver and kidneys from damage while relaxing nerve endings for eased detox symptoms. The peel also provides room-temperature stable vitamin C to facilitate metal excretion. Simply add 2 strips of fresh orange peel or ¼ teaspoon of dried peel to the tea 5 minutes before drinking.

Enjoy this refreshing cilantro, chlorella, and orange peel tea daily for 2-4 weeks to facilitate the safe elimination of potentially toxic heavy metals from the body. Time your initial rounds during warmer months for easier iced tea drinking since adequate daily fluid is crucial to flush the released metals. Listen to your body during the process and cut back as needed if any detox symptoms arise. With plans for heavy metal testing before and after your efforts, you can measure your success. Then repeat periodic gentle detoxes twice annually to limit ongoing heavy metal exposure threats.

Digestive Cleanser - Senna, Peppermint & Fennel Tea

A congested, compromised digestive system underlies many health issues. When the gut cannot properly break down foods, absorb nutrients, and eliminate wastes, toxic residues recirculate through the body causing dysfunction. Periodic cleansing of the digestive tract provides a reset. Key herbs that stimulate digestion and bowel movements while soothing the gut include senna leaf, peppermint, and fennel seed. Brewed together as a tea, they offer a gentle cleanse for the entire digestive system.

Senna leaf is the primary herb in this digestive cleanser tea. A member of the legume family, senna contains unique glycosides called sennosides that stimulate contractions in the smooth muscles of the colon. This increases motility to promote bowel movements and the elimination of waste and toxins from the digestive tract. Senna has been used medicinally for centuries as a natural laxative. It is considered very safe and non-habit forming when used appropriately.

For the tea, use 1 teaspoon of dried senna leaves or pods per cup of water. Steep the tea covered for 10-15 minutes before drinking to allow the sennosides to infuse. Senna gives the tea a slightly bitter, grassy taste. You can brew it overnight on very low heat to maximize extraction. Drink 1 cup of senna tea in the evening before bedtime as it can take 6-12 hours to produce an effect. Adjust the amount based on your individual response. Do not take senna longer than 1-2 weeks at a time and allow equal rest periods between use.
Peppermint nicely compliments senna in this digestive cleanser tea thanks to its carminative properties that help relieve bloating and gas. The menthol and volatile oil in peppermint relax the muscles of the intestinal tract to facilitate the movement and release of gas that can cause discomfort. Peppermint also alleviates abdominal cramps and nausea which can be associated with cleansing protocols. Its pleasant taste and aroma aid digestion.

Add 1 teaspoon dried peppermint leaf per cup of the senna tea. Steep for 10-15 minutes to allow both herbs to infuse before drinking 1 cup about an hour before bedtime. The cooling peppermint balances the warming senna leaf. You can also make a diluted peppermint tea separately to sip after meals during cleanses to ease any mild indigestion or gas pains that arise. Peppermint is very gentle and safe to use regularly for digestive problems.

The third herb in this tea, fennel seed, harmonizes beautifully with senna and peppermint to relax the gut, reduce inflammation, and enhance cleansing. Fennel seeds contain anethole, a phytoestrogen that eases gastrointestinal cramping, bloating, and inflammation. This allows for freer flow through the colon. Fennel also boosts bile production to improve digestion and deliver immune cells to the intestines. The licorice-like sweetness of fennel balances the other herbs nicely.

Add ½ teaspoon of fennel seeds per cup of hot water along with the senna leaves and peppermint leaves. Allow the tea to steeply cover for 10-15 minutes to develop the full flavor and aroma before drinking 1 cup before bedtime. Fennel is extremely gentle and safe even for regular use. You can also brew a larger batch of the digestive tea formula and drink it throughout the day in 1 cup increments if desired. Be sure to stagger consumption with meals however for optimal benefit.

This trifecta digestive cleanser tea harnessing senna, peppermint, and fennel works with your body's natural rhythms and processes to clear congestion and stagnation from the intestines. You can incorporate a 1-2 week cycle of this tea as part of any healthy cleanse or detox program for the best results. Pay attention to your body's signals, stay well hydrated between doses, and allow rest when needed during digestive cleansing periods. With this herbal tea trio, you can reset your digestive function periodically and maintain a healthy gut.

Chapter 8

Sleep Inducer: Chamomile, Passionflower and Lavender Tea

As the sun begins to set and the day winds down, our bodies naturally start to prepare for rest. But sometimes our busy lives and anxious minds keep us from easily drifting off to sleep. A nice cup of relaxing herbal tea can help pave the way for restful slumber. This Sleep Inducer tea combines chamomile, passionflower, and lavender - three herbs renowned for their sleep-promoting properties.

Chamomile is likely one of the most well-known sleepytime teas. This humble little white-petaled flower contains apigenin, an antioxidant flavonoid that binds to benzodiazepine receptors in the brain. These receptors are targeted by drugs used to treat anxiety and insomnia. Apigenin has a mild sedative effect, helping calm the mind and relax the nerves. Multiple studies have found chamomile tea can reduce anxiety and improve sleep quality. Its soothing nature makes it an excellent bedtime brew.

Passionflower is another herb traditionally used for its soothing, sleep-enhancing qualities. It contains compounds like harmala alkaloids that exert a sedative effect on the central nervous system. The flavonoids in passionflower have anti-anxiety, antispasmodic, and analgesic effects. Clinical trials have shown drinking passionflower tea before bed can help increase sleep time and quality. It's especially helpful for those who have trouble quitting their thoughts at night.

The sweet floral aroma of lavender is synonymous with relaxation. Linalool and linalyl acetate are two terpenes abundant in lavender that have sedative properties. Animal studies show lavender extracts increase time spent in deep, slow-wave sleep. Lavender's fragrance alone has a calming effect, lowering heart rate and blood pressure. Sipping lavender tea while soaking in a warm bath is a wonderful pre-bedtime ritual to unwind both body and mind.

This herbal blend takes advantage of the complementary effects of chamomile, passionflower, and lavender to promote tranquility and sleep. Chamomile calms the nerves, passionflower quiets the mind's chatter, and lavender casts a relaxing aroma to help you drift off to dreamland with ease. The ingredients work synergistically to relieve anxiety, muscular tension, and insomnia. It's a healthy, natural solution for when you're struggling to fall asleep.

To make Sleep Inducer tea:

Ingredients:

1 tablespoon dried chamomile flowers
1 tablespoon dried passion flower
½ tablespoon dried lavender buds
8 ounces hot water
Steep the chamomile, passionflower, and lavender in hot water for 5-7 minutes. Strain tea into a mug. Sip slowly 30-60 minutes before bed. Make a larger batch and refrigerate leftover tea to reheat as needed. Drink every night for the best effects. Can be enjoyed with a bit of honey or lemon to taste.

This relaxing herbal tea is safe to consume every night to unwind before bed. For most people chamomile, passionflower and lavender do not cause any side effects or morning grogginess. Those taking sedatives or antidepressants should check with their doctor before using them. Pregnant or nursing mothers should also consult their physician first.

Settling down for the night with a hot cup of Sleep Inducer tea is a soothing ritual to relax both the body and mind. The combination of chamomile, passionflower, and lavender works gently to relieve worries, quiet your thoughts, and invite restful sleep. Sip slowly and breathe deeply as you drink. Let the floral flavors and aromas wash your stress away. Within 30-60 minutes you'll start to feel pleasantly drowsy. Sleep will become easier as your muscles unwind and anxieties fade. Soon you'll be drifting off to sleep peacefully, ready to wake refreshed in the morning.

Rest Easy: Valerian and Hops Nightcap Tea

If you're someone who struggles with falling asleep, staying asleep or getting quality sleep, this Rest Easy tea made with valerian and hops is the perfect natural solution. Valerian has been used for centuries as a sleep aid. Modern research confirms what traditional herbalists have long known - valerian is one of nature's best remedies for insomnia. When combined with the calming qualities of hops, this tea promotes deep, restorative sleep so you can wake up refreshed.

Valerian contains over 150 active components, including valerenic acid and valerenol. These compounds interact with GABA receptors and inhibit enzyme activity in the brain, working as a mild sedative. Multiple clinical studies substantiate valerian's effectiveness in improving sleep quality and reducing the time it takes to fall asleep.

It helps regulate sleep cycles, allowing you to spend more time in slow wave and rapid eye movement (REM) sleep.

In addition to its sedative qualities, valerian has anxiolytic effects to relieve stress and nervous restlessness that can interfere with sleep. The valepotriates and sesquiterpenes in valerian increase the availability of GABA in the brain, lowering anxiety levels. The result is a profound calming effect perfect for nighttime. Valerian also has hypotensive action to relieve muscle tension and pain that can disrupt sleep.

Hops, best known for their use in beer brewing, impart a wonderfully relaxing quality to this nighttime tea. The compounds myrcene, humulene and xanthohumol contribute to hops' sedative nature, working in harmony with valerian. Hops increase non-REM sleep time and induce drowsiness by modulating GABA neurotransmission. The flavonoids in hops also have anti-anxiety benefits to further promote tranquility and sleep.

This dynamic duo makes falling asleep effortlessly easy. The valerian relieves worry and nervous unrest, while the hops banish muscle tension and pain. Together these herbs calm both the mind and body, releasing you into a deep, peaceful slumber. Regular use can help correct insomnia and improve sleep quality. Wake up feeling well-rested and refreshed.

To make Rest Easy tea:

Ingredients:

1 tablespoon dried valerian root
1 teaspoon dried hops strobiles
8 ounces hot water

Place valerian root and hops in a tea infuser. Steep in hot water for 5-10 minutes. Strain tea into a mug. Drink 30-60 minutes before bedtime. Can be enjoyed with a teaspoon of honey if desired.

For best results, drink a cup nightly 1 hour before bedtime. This tea is safe for regular consumption for healthy adults. Those taking benzodiazepines or sedative medications should exercise caution. Pregnant and nursing women should also avoid valerian. Do not use this tea alongside alcohol or other sleep aids.

Set aside all screens and distractions when you sit down with your bedtime tea. Sip slowly and focus on the earthy, hoppy flavor. Feel the warmth relax your body as the herbs soothe your mind. Anxiety and worry melt away as your muscles loosen. Within an hour you'll be lulled into a deep, tranquil sleep. Sleep soundly through the night and awake rest. With regular use, valerian and hops can help correct chronic insomnia for good. You'll look forward to relaxing with a hot cup of Rest Easy tea as part of your nightly wind-down ritual.

Calming Magnolia and Jujube Zizyphus Tea

Do you have trouble silencing your thoughts when it's time for bed? Does your mind race keep you awake far longer than you'd like? Say goodbye to restless nights with this Calming Magnolia and Jujube Zizyphus tea. Combining the ancient Chinese herbs magnolia and jujube dates, it eases anxiety and unwinds an overactive mind for restful sleep all night long.

Magnolia bark, known as Hou Po in Traditional Chinese Medicine, has a long history of use for treating stress, anxiety, and insomnia. It contains magnolol and honokiol, two active compounds that exert significant anti-anxiety and sleep-promoting effects. Studies show magnolia bark alleviates psychological stress while increasing GABA activity in the brain. GABA is the primary inhibitory neurotransmitter responsible for calming nervous activity. With regular use, magnolia bark can help rebalance GABA levels to reduce anxiety and promote tranquility.

Jujube dates, or Ziziphus jujuba, have mild sedative properties to complement magnolia bark. Jujube is packed with antioxidants like flavonoids, phenolic acids, and polysaccharides that protect the brain and encourage restful sleep. It supports healthy neurotransmitter production, including serotonin which regulates sleep cycles, and melatonin which controls our circadian rhythms. Jujube also boosts immune function to help fight off stress-induced illness.

Together, magnolia bark and jujube work synergistically to rid both mind and body of tension. Magnolia calms thoughts and alleviates anxiety, while jujube boosts mood, immunity, and sleep-wake cycles. Sipping this tea naturally relaxes the nervous system. Racing thoughts smooth to stillness. Shoulders soften as muscles relax. Its mildly sedative effect helps you easily drift into tranquil slumber.

Calming Magnolia and Jujube Zizyphus Tea

Do you have trouble silencing your thoughts when it's time for bed? Does your mind race keep you awake far longer than you'd like? Say goodbye to restless nights with this Calming Magnolia and Jujube Zizyphus tea. Combining the ancient Chinese herbs magnolia and jujube dates, it eases anxiety and unwinds an overactive mind for restful sleep all night long.

Magnolia bark, known as Hou Po in Traditional Chinese Medicine, has a long history of use for treating stress, anxiety and insomnia. It contains magnolol and honokiol, two active compounds that exert significant anti-anxiety and sleep-promoting effects. Studies show magnolia bark alleviates psychological stress while increasing GABA activity in the brain. GABA is the primary inhibitory neurotransmitter responsible for calming nervous activity. With regular use, magnolia bark can help rebalance GABA levels to reduce anxiety and promote tranquility.

Jujube dates, or Ziziphus jujuba, have mild sedative properties to complement magnolia bark. Jujube is packed with antioxidants like flavonoids, phenolic acids, and polysaccharides that protect the brain and encourage restful sleep. It supports healthy neurotransmitter production, including serotonin which regulates sleep cycles, and melatonin which controls our circadian rhythms. Jujube also boosts immune function to help fight off stress-induced illness.

Together, magnolia bark and jujube work synergistically to rid both mind and body of tension. Magnolia calms thoughts and alleviates anxiety, while jujube boosts mood, immunity, and sleep-wake cycles. Sipping this tea naturally relaxes the nervous system. Racing thoughts smooth to stillness. Shoulders soften as muscles relax. Its mildly sedative effect helps you easily drift into tranquil slumber.

Dream Awakener: Mugwort, Rose, and Flaxseed Tea

Do you wish you could remember your dreams better or have more vivid, intense dream experiences? Tap into the dream-enhancing powers of mugwort, rose, and flaxseed with this Night Awakener tea. Sipping this herbal blend before bed can help stimulate dream recall, intensify dream color and imagery, and induce lucid dreaming.

Mugwort has a long history in folklore for its dream-influencing properties. Used for centuries in shamanic rituals, this aromatic herb contains compounds like thujone that interact with GABA receptors in the brain. This activity leads to heightened imagination and more memorable, meaningful dreams. Studies confirm mugwort increases dream activity and recall upon awakening.

Adding rose petals augments mugwort's oneiric effects. Rose is high in antioxidants like lycopene and vitamin C which protect the brain while you sleep and dream. It contains nerol and geraniol, aromatic compounds that help relax the body and stimulate the mind's creativity. Rose essential oil has even been shown in sleep studies to increase time spent in REM when vivid dreaming occurs.

Nutty, earthy flaxseed rounds out the trio. A good source of sleep-supportive nutrients like tryptophan and magnesium, flaxseed helps regulate circadian rhythms and melatonin secretion. The healthy fats in flaxseed, like omega-3 alpha-linolenic acid, also boost neurotransmitter activity for optimal dream state benefits.

Together, these herbs unlock your dreamscape for dazzling nightly adventures. As you slumber deeply, mugwort kindles your subconscious imagination and heightens dream intensity. Rose amplifies imagery and fuels creativity. Flaxseed nourishes brain health to support REM sleep. Upon waking, dreams remain vivid in technicolor detail. You may even experience moments of lucidity in which you become aware it's a dream.

This tea is safe for regular use unless you have an estrogen-sensitive condition like breast cancer. Avoid use during pregnancy and breastfeeding. Those on psychiatric medications should consult their doctor first.

For best dream-enhancing results:

Drink 1 cup about 30 minutes before bedtime
Keep a dream journal on your nightstand to record dreams upon waking
Repeat affirmations before bed such as "I will remember my dreams"
Soon your dream world will transform into an expansive landscape for your imagination to play. Nightly escapades bring new self-awareness and creativity into your waking life. Sweet dreams!

Slip into vivid alternate realms each night with a cup of Dream Awakener tea before bed. This unique blend of mugwort, rose and flaxseed kindles your imagination for dazzling dreamscapes. As you prepare for sleep, brew a cup to open your mind's eye to nocturnal adventures.

Mugwort's mystique traces back centuries for its supernatural effects on dreams. Called the "dream sage", mugwort contains compounds like thujone that interact with GABA receptors in the brain. This activity inhibits certain neurotransmitters, leading to a hypnagogic state perfect for lucid dreaming.

Modern research confirms mugwort's dream-enhancing qualities. Regularly sipping mugwort tea dramatically improves dream recall and intensity of imagery. Under Mugwort's influence, ordinary dreams transform into highly sensorial experiences. You may encounter deceased loved ones, receive creative insights, or realize you're dreaming while asleep. Lucid dreams are like virtual reality where you control the scenarios.

Adding vivid rose petals enhances mugwort's oneiric magic. Rose contains nerol and geraniol, aromatic compounds that calm the body while stimulating the mind's creativity. Rich in antioxidants like lycopene and vitamin C, rose safeguards the brain during your slumber. Studies also demonstrate that rose essential oil heightens REM sleep when dreaming occurs.

Nutty flaxseed rounds out this trinity, providing sleep-supportive nutrients like tryptophan, magnesium, and thiamine. The healthy fats in flaxseed boost neurotransmitters for optimal dream state benefits. Grounding flax brings your intentions to reality so you recall messages from your dreams upon waking.

To prepare for revelatory rest:

Journal dreams in the morning
Set intention before bed to remember dreams
Repeat mantras like "I recall my dreams"
Try B6, B12, or 5-HTP supplements
Record your dreams immediately after waking, even fragmentary bits and pieces. Use journals, voice memos, or apps like DreamMapper to help cement recall. Notice dream signs like animals, cars, or teeth that may indicate you're dreaming. Doing regular reality checks when awake teaches your mind to recognize dreams.

Each night as you sip this tea, focus your thoughts on your intention to remember dreams and sleep well. Dim the lights and remove distractions to enter a relaxed state as the herbs take effect. Slip into bed peacefully, allowing your consciousness to expand as you drift into slumber.

Upon waking, lingering in a hypnopompic state can help access dream memories before they fade. Stay relaxed with your eyes closed, retracing your steps backward through dream space. Jot down notes and record dreams in your journal before getting out of bed. Over time, regular dream journaling first thing in the morning will dramatically improve recall.

Dream Awakener tea opens portals to exotic dream realms each night. Your inner landscape will flourish with mugwort's lush imagery, rose's divine creativity, and flax's grounding wisdom. Charting your dreams reveals recurring places, people, and scenarios that provide insight into your emotional world. This tea also boosts confidence in trusting your intuition derived from nocturnal inner work.

Tension Tamer: Lemongrass, Skullcap, and Kava Tea

Does your mind feel overloaded and your body tense after a stressful day? Having trouble unwinding when it's time for bed? Soothe your worries away with a hot cup of Tension Tamer tea. Featuring lemongrass, skullcap, and kava, this relaxing blend melts away the mental and physical burdens of the day for a peaceful slumber.

Tropical, citrusy lemongrass is renowned for its anxiety-relieving qualities. Studies demonstrate oral dosages of lemongrass essential oil relieve stress and lower cortisol levels. Lemongrass contains the flavonoids orientin and vicenin which exert sedative effects on the central nervous system. This helps quiet mental chatter that keeps you tossing and turning into the night.

Skullcap is a minty North American herb traditionally used to alleviate nervous tension, anxiety, and muscular tightness. It contains antioxidants like quercetin along with skullcap flavones that reduce inflammation and nourish the nervous system. Skullcap increases GABA activity to promote calm. It also relieves muscle spasms, headaches, and teeth grinding caused by excessive stress.

Kava kava is a Polynesian herb that has significant anti-anxiety and muscle relaxant effects perfect for unwinding in the evening. The active compounds called kavalactones reduce excitability in the brain while promoting muscle relaxation. Research confirms kava as a non-addictive sleep aid that can help you fall asleep faster and sleep more soundly.

Sipping this soothing blend before bed helps melt away the leftover tension of your day. Lemongrass and skullcap work together to relieve anxiety and quiet mental chatter. Kava kava loosens tight muscles and calms restless legs. Within 30-60 minutes you'll feel relaxed and ready for sleep. Enjoy this tea nightly to reduce stress and restore healthy sleep rhythms.

To make Tension Tamer tea:

1 tablespoon dried lemongrass
1 tablespoon dried skullcap
1 tablespoon kava root powder
8 ounces hot water
Steep the lemongrass, skullcap, and kava powder in hot water for 5-7 minutes. Strain and drink 30-60 minutes before bedtime. Add lemon or honey to taste if desired.

Set aside digital devices and distractions to fully relax as you slowly sip this tea. With each swallow feel the herbs release the accumulated tension of your day. Muscles soften as your mind empties of worry. Soon you'll melt into the comfort of your bed, drifting into tranquil slumber. Wake restored and ready for a new day.

At the end of a stressful day when your mind is overloaded and body tense, this relaxing Tension Tamer tea is just what you need. As soon as you get home, put on the kettle and begin your evening wind-down ritual with a hot cup of this soothing blend.

Lemongrass, skullcap, and kava kava work synergistically to melt away the mental and physical burdens of your day. Light, lemony lemongrass calms worries and quiets racing thoughts. Skullcap alleviates nervous tension, anxiety, and tight muscles. And kava kava's kavalactones provide potent anxiolytic and muscle relaxant effects to unwind completely.

Together, these herbs help smooth the transition from a busy day to a tranquil evening. The bright, grassy flavor of lemongrass mingles with earthy skullcap and rich kava for a complex soothing cup. Fill your kitchen with this tea's comforting aromas as you slowly sip, consciously releasing the accumulated stress of your day with each swallow.

Over the next 30-60 minutes you'll feel your shoulders soften as your mind empties of repetitive thoughts. Let the medicinal wisdom of the herbs seep into every cell, relaxing body and spirit. Muscles unwind as a sense of calm washes over you. Allow any irritation or anxiety to dissolve, making space for the tranquility that emerges.

This evening ritual cleanses your palate after a long day of busyness, letting your highest self shine through. Reflect on any insights or inspiration that surface as you become fully immersed in the present moment. Feel deeply grateful for the opportunity to relax and replenish your energy. Sleep will come easier tonight, letting you awake refreshed for a new day.

Keep a batch of Tension Tamer tea on hand for stressful days when you need to unwind. The earthy aromas and medicinal flavors are deeply grounding. Mindfully prepare your cup, then sit and sip without any distractions. Make space for stillness as the herbs work their magic, leaving you relaxed, renewed, and ready for restful sleep.

Morning Mover: Dandelion, Ginger, and Lemon Balm Tea

Rise and shine with this refreshing and energizing Morning Mover tea. Featuring dandelion root, ginger, and lemon balm, this lively blend stimulates digestion, boosts metabolism and weakens your senses first thing in the morning. Start your day off right with a cup to help you feel bright, alert, and ready to take on anything.

Dandelion root is a powerfully cleansing herb that supports detoxification and healthy digestion. It stimulates bile production and gastrointestinal motility to relieve sluggish bowels. The bitter compounds taraxacin and taraxacin provide mild laxative effects. Dandelion root is also a rich source of the antioxidant beta-carotene which gives this tea a bright golden color.

The fresh flavor of ginger adds warming spice to wake up your palate. Gingerols and shogaols give ginger its zippy zing, which stokes your digestive fire in the morning. Ginger boosts circulation and contains anti-inflammatory compounds called gingerols that energize the body. Studies show ginger's aroma can even improve mood, reaction time, and focus first thing in the morning.

Rounding out this blend is lemon balm, a minty lemon herb traditionally used for its uplifting, revitalizing properties. It has an invigorating citrus aroma that stimulates the senses. Rosmarinic acid and flavonoids give lemon balm potent antioxidant activity to protect cells from early morning oxidative damage. Studies also demonstrate it can significantly improve mood and mental performance.

Sipping this vibrant tea first thing in the morning will get your day off to an optimal start. Dandelion root cleanses and stimulates digestion and metabolism. Ginger warms and energizes your body while improving concentration. Lemon balm lifts your mood and sharpens your mind. Within 30 minutes you'll feel awake, focused, and ready to take on the day!

To make Morning Mover tea:

1 tablespoon dried dandelion root
1 teaspoon grated fresh ginger
1 teaspoon dried lemon balm
8 ounces hot water
Steep the herbs in hot water for 5-7 minutes. Strain and sweeten with a teaspoon of honey if desired. Drink 1 cup every morning on an empty stomach.

Set your intention to have an energized, productive day as you slowly savor your morning cup of Morning Mover. Feel the dandelion root clear stagnation as ginger stokes your inner fire. Lemon balm brightens your mood and energizes your mind. You'll be ready to seize the day with gusto!

This lively blend of dandelion, ginger, and lemon balm is the perfect way to start your morning off right. As the first rays of sunlight filter through your window, brew up a hot cup of Morning Mover tea to gently awaken your body and mind.

The dynamic combination of herbs in this tea supports healthy digestion, circulation, metabolism, and energy levels to get you energized for the day ahead. Dandelion root kickstarts your gastrointestinal system with its bitter principles and mild laxative effects. The bright, golden root stimulates the release of bile from the gallbladder to promote fat digestion and keep food moving smoothly through your intestines. Regular morning doses of dandelion can help relieve occasional constipation while cleansing the liver.

Tangy ginger adds its warming magic to get your blood pumping and metabolism fueled. Gingerol, the main bioactive compound in ginger, gives it that spicy-sweet zing that tingles your taste buds awake. This potent phytochemical has impressive antioxidant and anti-inflammatory effects to support whole-body health. Ginger also contains essential oils like zingiberene that help reduce nausea, bloating, gas, and other tummy troubles. Sipping ginger tea first thing gently stimulates digestion and circulation to start your day off comfortably.

Uplifting lemon balm completes the trio with its fresh herbaceous flavor and wild lemon scent. Abundant in antioxidant, and anti-inflammatory flavonoids, lemon balm lifts your spirits while calming nervous tension that can accumulate overnight. Studies show it can significantly improve mood and mental alertness in the morning. The citrusy aroma helps stimulate your senses so you feel awake and ready to take on the day.

Set your intention the night before to rise early enough to slowly savor this medicinal brew. Allow at least 15-30 minutes to mindfully drink your cup of Morning Mover tea in the quiet morning stillness. Breathe deeply to take in the aroma of lemon balm's volatile oils. Feel the comforting warmth spread through your belly as ginger kindles your inner fire. Absorb dandelion's sunny vibes as vital energy flows through your body.

Step outside into the fresh morning air after finishing your tea, feeling rejuvenated and inspired for the day ahead. Carry that bright, focused energy with you as you mindfully move through your morning routine. You'll be amazed how a simple cup of herbs can set the tone for an energized, productive day. Make Morning Mover tea part of your regular ritual so you can greet each new sunrise with clarity and joy.

Chapter 9

Menstrual Comfort: Raspberry Leaf, Cinnamon and Ginger Tea

Many women experience menstrual discomfort including cramps, bloating, and heavy bleeding. Herbal teas can provide relief by relaxing uterine muscles, acting as anti-inflammatories, and providing nourishing minerals. Raspberry leaf is one of the most popular herbs for menstrual health. It contains fragrance, a uterine tonic that relaxes and tones the uterus, reducing painful cramps and spasms. Raspberry leaf is also high in iron, an important mineral for replacing blood lost during menstruation. Cinnamon adds warming and anti-inflammatory properties to raspberry leaf tea, further relaxing uterine muscles and easing cramps. Ginger is another warming herb that reduces inflammation, gastrointestinal upset, and nausea.

To make this herbal tea, steep 1-2 teaspoons of dried raspberry leaf and a pinch of cinnamon and ginger in 8 ounces of boiling water for 5-10 minutes. Strain and drink up to 3 cups daily during menstruation. The tea has a pleasant, fruity taste. Some women begin drinking the tea daily during the entire month leading up to their period to maximize benefits. Raspberry leaf does not interact negatively with medications and is safe for most women. Those with heavy menstrual bleeding should use raspberry leaf under the guidance of a herbalist or naturopathic doctor.

This herbal tea blend provides a safe, effective option for dealing with the discomfort many women experience during their cycles. The tannins and fragrance in raspberry leaf relieve cramps by gently relaxing the smooth muscle of the uterus. Cinnamon adds antioxidant, anti-inflammatory, and antispasmodic properties to further aid cramping. Ginger reduces inflammation, warms the body, and minimizes nausea. Enjoying a warm cup of this herbal infusion makes menstruation more comfortable.

Fertili-Tea: Red Raspberry, Red Clover, and Nettle Tea

Trying to conceive can be an emotional rollercoaster full of hope, disappointment, and frustration. Herbs that support healthy fertility can help optimize the chances of pregnancy naturally in women without medical fertility issues. Red raspberry leaf tones the uterine muscles, improving the chance of conception and healthy implantation of an embryo. It also provides key nutrients such as vitamins C, E, A, and B complex, as well as minerals like calcium, iron, and potassium. Red clover blossoms contain isoflavones that mimic estrogen, helping regulate hormonal balance, promote ovulation, and increase cervical mucus. Stinging nettle leaf is mineral-rich, providing iron, chlorophyll, vitamins C and K, calcium, and potassium. It reduces inflammation, balances hormones, and promotes uterine health.

To make this fertility-boosting blend, steep 1 teaspoon each of dried red raspberry leaf, red clover blossoms, and nettle leaf in 8 ounces of boiling water for 5-10 minutes. Strain and drink up to 3 cups daily. Enjoy the mild, slightly sweet taste of this nourishing infusion. Use for 3-6 months prior to trying to conceive and throughout the first trimester of pregnancy to support implantation and fetal development. These herbs are safe for most women, but those with estrogen-sensitive conditions should consult their healthcare provider before using red clover.

Trying for a baby is an emotional, demanding journey. Using herbs to optimize uterine health and hormonal balance improves the chances of conception naturally. Red raspberry leaf tones the uterus, red clover enhances cervical mucus and regulates hormones, and stinging nettle provides minerals and reduces inflammation. Sipping this herbal tea daily helps create a hospitable environment for new life to take root and grow.

Lady's Mantle and Spearmint Hormone Balancer Tea

Hormonal fluctuations are an inevitable part of being a woman. But when hormones are severely out of balance, they can wreak havoc on physical and emotional health. Symptoms like infertility, acne, excessive hair growth, weight gain, headaches, anxiety, fatigue, and irregular cycles steal joy and productivity. Pharmaceuticals provide an option for regulating hormones, but herbal teas can gently restore balance without completely disrupting the body's delicate hormonal ecosystem. Lady's mantle and spearmint make an effective pairing that minimizes the highs and lows to help you feel like yourself again.

Lady's mantle contains astringent tannins, soothing volatile oils, and anti-inflammatory flavonoids. This herb minimizes menstrual bleeding when it becomes heavy or prolonged. It also relaxes uterine muscle spasms to decrease menstrual cramps. The key medicinal actions of lady's mantle on the reproductive system are:

Astringent: Constricts tissues and reduces secretions

Anti-inflammatory: Calms inflammation
Vulnerary: Promotes wound healing
Sedative: Relaxes muscular tension and spasms
These properties help normalize uterine bleeding while easing pain and spasms. Lady's mantle also regulates the hypothalamic-pituitary-ovarian axis which controls the menstrual cycle. It provides restorative, normalizing actions on the uterus and ovaries as a "female tonic".

In addition to benefiting reproductive health, lady's mantle extracts exhibit antioxidant and anti-diabetic activities. The herb's anti-inflammatory and astringent effects likely calm inflammation and stabilize blood sugar. Lady's mantle is an excellent herb for women with menstrual problems linked to hormone imbalance, such as endometriosis or uterine fibroids. It reduces bleeding and cramping while gently tonifying the reproductive system.

Menopause Cooler: Sage, Black Cohosh, and Dong Quai Tea

Menopause heralds a new beginning filled with promise. But before entering this liberating stage, women must navigate an often-turbulent transition marked by hormonal fluctuations. Hot flashes, insomnia, fatigue, vaginal dryness, mood swings, and other unpleasant symptoms commonly disrupt daily life throughout perimenopause and menopause. Pharmaceutical hormones provide one option for relieving these effects, but natural herbal teas offer a more balanced approach.Sage, black cohosh, and dong quai make an effective trio for easing menopause symptoms. Together they calm hot flashes, improve sleep quality, stabilize mood, increase vaginal secretions, and support bone health. Let's explore the therapeutic actions of each herb:

Sage:

Contains antioxidant flavonoids that regulate neurotransmitters
Lower the incidence of hot flashes
Inhibit excessive sweating
Improves cognitive function
Boost mood and ease irritability
Black Cohosh:

Phytoestrogens reduce hot flashes and night sweats
Relieves anxiety and irritability, mood swings
Aids sleep quality
Eases aching muscles and joints
Protects bone mineral density
Dong Quai:

Regulates estrogen levels
Improves vaginal dryness
Reduces hot flashes
Lessens mood swings
Supports bone strength
Steep 1 teaspoon each of dried sage, black cohosh root, and dong quai root in 8 ounces freshly boiled water for 10 minutes. Drink 1-2 cups of tea daily. The savory, earthy blend provides a nutritive beverage enjoyed by women across cultures for centuries. Monitor your symptoms to determine the optimal dosage and frequency.

Sage and dong quai are quite safe for extended use but do not take black cohosh for longer than 6 months at a time. Consult your healthcare provider before using black cohosh if you have liver problems. Discontinue any herb that causes nausea, headache, dizziness or upset stomach.

Rather than abruptly cutting off estrogen production, this tea helps your body gracefully transition to a new homeostasis. Finally bid farewell to the hot flashes, irritability, and sleepless nights of hormonal upheaval. Sip your way through menopause and beyond with nature's wisdom in each cup.

Nursing Tea: Fennel, Fenugreek, and Blessed Thistle Tea

Breastfeeding provides the perfect nutrition for babies to thrive. It offers unique benefits like boosting immunity, reducing infections, and fostering a special bond between mother and child. However, many new mothers struggle to produce enough breast milk to meet their baby's needs. Before turning to formula, herbs provide a natural way to increase milk supply. Certain herbs called galactagogues safely promote lactation when incorporated into a nursing mother's diet.

Fennel seed, fenugreek seed, and blessed thistle are three excellent galactagogues that stimulate milk production by mimicking estrogen's effects on breast tissue. Together they help ensure your baby receives the nutrients only your milk can provide. Let's explore how each herb in this blend supports a healthy milk supply:

Fennel Seeds:

Increase prolactin, the hormone regulating milk synthesis
Regulate menstrual cycles which optimizes postpartum milk production
Improve milk flow, volume, and fat content
Reduce inflammation which can inhibit milk ejection
Relieve colic, gas, and diarrhea in breastfed infants
Fenugreek Seeds:

Contain diosgenin which amplifies milk duct development and activity

Boost levels of prolactin along with growth hormones important for milk quality

Increase milk volume by stimulating sweat gland activity in breasts

Improve milk composition with higher vitamin and mineral levels

Reduce mastitis by clearing clogged milk ducts

Blessed Thistle:

Stimulates secretion of gastric juices to optimize nutrient absorption for milk

Contains antioxidants that remove toxins and boost immune health in mother

Astringent and anti-inflammatory effects increase overall milk supply

Relieve indigestion and support liver health in postpartum mothers

Steep 1 teaspoon each of dried fennel, fenugreek, and blessed thistle seeds in 8 ounces of freshly boiled water for 10 minutes. Strain and drink 2-3 cups daily. The earthy, subtly licorice-like tea is mild enough to enjoy long-term while nursing. Monitor your baby's output and weight gain to determine the right dosage for your needs.

These herbs have been used safely for many years to support breastfeeding, but discuss taking galactagogues with your doctor or lactation consultant first. Start with 1 cup per day and watch for any signs of digestive upset or allergic reaction in your baby before increasing intake. Never take fenugreek while pregnant - it can stimulate uterine contractions.

You are giving your infant the greatest gift by nourishing them with your milk. Herbal teas make sure your supply keeps up with their growing appetite. Sip this brew often so your angel continues getting all the benefits of your liquid gold.

Common Challenges When Breastfeeding and Their Solutions

Breastfeeding provides the perfect food designed specifically to help your baby thrive. However, many new mothers encounter challenges that can disrupt the nursing process if not addressed. Here are some of the most common hurdles and tips to overcome them:

Cramp Crusher: Wild Yam, Valerian, and Jamaican Dogwood Tea

Menstrual cramps can range from mildly annoying to completely debilitating for many women. Cramps stem from prostaglandins triggering uterine muscle spasms during menstruation. For some, the abdominal cramping and lower back pain cause misery for several days each month, leading to lost productivity and social isolation.

Over-the-counter painkillers provide temporary relief but can cause side effects with long-term use. Herbal teas offer fast-acting natural cramp relief without risks by relaxing smooth muscle tissue, reducing inflammation, and easing anxiety associated with pain. Wild yam, valerian, and Jamaican dogwood make an effective combination.

Wild yam contains antispasmodic saponins that quickly relieve uterine and intestinal cramping. The herb contains diosgenin, a phytoestrogen that reduces muscle spasms in the uterus, ovary, and GI tract. Diosgenin also blocks prostaglandin synthesis to decrease period pain.

Valerian reduces muscle spasms and anxiety that can exacerbate cramps. It contains valerenic acids and valepotriates that bind to GABA receptors and serotonin. This action reduces nerve excitability and tension in the uterine muscles. Valerian also lowers prostaglandin production.

Jamaican dogwood acts as a sedative and analgesic to relax the body and minimize pain perception. It relieves spasms and discomfort without suppressing the central nervous system as much as pharmaceutical sedatives. The herb also reduces anxiety which can heighten the feeling of pain.

Chapter 10

Herbal Teas for Men's Health

Men's health concerns are often overlooked or seen as taboo to discuss openly. However, issues like prostate health, sexual function, stress levels, and urinary flow are important to address. Making simple changes like incorporating targeted herbal teas into your routine can provide noticeable improvements.

Herbal teas offer a comforting, ritualistic way to hydrate while steeping your body in plant-based compounds. The herbal infusion releases active constituents over a 30+ minute period, allowing for gradual absorption. This makes teas an optimal delivery method for botanical supplements. The act of slowly sipping a hot cup of tea also promotes relaxation during hectic modern life.

When harnessing herbs, quality matters. Seek out organic, ethically wild-harvested, or biodynamically grown herbs from reputable sources. Store teas in a cool, dark place to preserve potency. Brewing with filtered, spring, or mineral water will limit unwanted chemicals while extracting the greatest benefits from the herbs. Avoid diluting efficacy by over-steeping. Follow preparation guidelines for optimal extraction.

The expansive world of herbal tea provides diverse options for men's health. From soothing prostates and enhancing libido to easing anxiety and supporting urinary flow, targeted teas offer natural solutions. Explore incorporating one or more of these restorative herbal teas into your routine.

Prostate Aid: Saw Palmetto, Stinging Nettle and Pygeum Tea

The prostate gland tends to enlarge in most men as they age, starting around age 40. This common, non-cancerous condition is known as benign prostatic hyperplasia (BPH). An enlarged prostate compressing the urethra can cause troubling urinary symptoms like reduced flow, hesitancy, frequent night urination, incontinence, and retention.

Saw palmetto, stinging nettle, and pygeum are three extensively researched herbs that have been shown to help relieve BPH symptoms. Combining all three into a tea provides synergistic prostate support.

More Herbal Teas for Men's Health

Discover more restorative herbal teas to incorporate into your daily ritual. Pay attention to your body's responses to identify which teas provide you the greatest benefits. Your ideal tea blends may vary day to day based on your changing health needs. Continue reading to learn about 10 more herbal teas for optimizing men's vitality.

Muscle Builder: Creatine and Cordyceps Tea

Active men looking to build lean muscle mass can benefit from herbal teas that supplement workout nutrition. Creatine and cordyceps are two supplements that help promote muscle growth and strength when combined with resistance training. Enjoy this tea daily for cumulative effects.

Creatine is a nitrogenous organic acid that occurs naturally in meat and fish. However, supplementing 5-10 grams of creatine monohydrate daily has been shown to significantly boost muscle mass and performance during high-intensity weight lifting. Luckily, creatine is also highly water soluble.

Dissolving creatine monohydrate powder in a hot cup of herbal tea is an easy way to ingest your daily creatine. This provides both hydration and supplementation in one warm, comforting beverage. Steeping with lemon can help break down the creatine for better absorption.

Adding cordyceps mushroom powder doubles the muscle-building potential. Cordyceps are revered in Traditional Chinese Medicine for enhancing vitality. Compounds like cordycepic acid and antioxidants give cordyceps anti-fatigue effects. Studies confirm cordyceps increase energy production, endurance, and exercise capacity.

Simply stir 1-2 teaspoons each of creatine and cordyceps mushroom powder into your favorite black, green, or herbal tea. Drink 1-2 cups daily for workout days to amplify your muscle-building results. Pair with a protein and carbohydrate-rich post-workout recovery meal.

Men's Health Herbal Tea Recipes

Now that we've covered a plethora of beneficial herbs for optimizing men's health in tea form, let's look at some blended recipes you can start brewing and enjoying today. Combining several synergistic herbs allows you to target multiple health goals in one cup.

Experiment with these recipes as a template for crafting your own custom daily brews.

Matcha Energy Tonic

This antioxidant-rich blend provides clean fuel for active lifestyles and razor-sharp mental performance.

Ingredients:

1 tsp Matcha green tea powder
½ tsp Rhodiola root powder
½ tsp Cordyceps mushroom powder
¼ tsp Cocoa nibs or raw cacao powder
1 cup hot filtered water
Dash of cinnamon
Optional: milk/milk alternative to taste
Instructions: Sift matcha powder through a small mesh strainer to avoid clumping. Add rhodiola, cordyceps, cacao nibs, and cinnamon to a mug. Pour a small amount of hot water over top and whisk vigorously with a frother or small whisk to form a paste. Add remaining water and continue whisking until foamy. Add milk/milk alternative if desired.

Benefits: This energizing brew provides a combination of adaptogens, antioxidants, and amino acids to lift mood, heighten focus, and power through your day. The mix of matcha, rhodiola, and cocoa provides a balanced energy lift without jitters.

Muscle Recovery Chai

Replenish nutrients and reduce inflammation after exercise with this spiced herbal infusion.

The Ultimate Tea Recipe Book

Ingredients:

1 black tea bag or 2 tsp loose tea
1 tsp Ashwagandha powder
1 tsp Creatine monohydrate powder
½ tsp Cinnamon chips or powder
¼ tsp Powdered ginger
¼ tsp Allspice
¼ tsp Cardamom pods, crushed
8 oz hot water or nut milk
Instructions: Combine all ingredients in a mug and pour hot water or steamed nut milk over top. Allow to steep for 5-10 minutes, then stir and enjoy. Sweeten lightly with honey if desired.

Benefits: Ashwagandha reduces cortisol and inflammation caused by strenuous workouts. Creatine aids muscle repair and growth. Anti-inflammatory spices like ginger, cinnamon, and allspice ease swollen muscles. Sip while refueling with protein and carbs.

Tranquility Prostate Tea

Soothe prostate swelling and urinary urgency with these cooling herbs.

Ingredients:

1 tbsp Saw Palmetto berries
1 tbsp Stinging Nettle leaf
1 tsp Parsley leaf
½ tsp Marshmallow root
½ tsp Elderberry
½ tsp Fennel seeds

1 cup boiling water
1 tsp raw honey (optional)
Instructions: Combine all herbs in a mug and pour boiling water over top. Allow to steep for at least 10 minutes before straining. Sweeten with honey if desired. Drink 1-2 times daily.

Benefits: Saw palmetto, stinging nettle, parsley, and marshmallow root work synergistically to reduce prostate inflammation and ease urinary discomfort. Elderberry and fennel provide additional antioxidant and anti-inflammatory effects.

Preparing and Enjoying Herbal Tea

Now that we've extensively covered specific herbs and blended recipes for optimizing men's health, let's look at some best practices for preparing and savoring your daily cups of tea. Proper methods for brewing and drinking herbal tea will help you derive maximum benefits from these healing botanicals.

Choosing Quality Ingredients
Organic, ethically wild-harvested, or biodynamically grown herbs from reputable sources ensure safety and potency. Seek out small-batch herbs instead of mass-produced ones. Check expiration dates and avoid faded, musty, or stale ingredients. Whole herbs retain potency better than pre-powdered. Store in sealed glass jars away from heat, air, and sunlight.

Double-check the safety of any herbs new to you, especially if on medications or with a medical condition. While most tea herbs are very safe, a small minority can interact with drugs or exacerbate health problems at high doses. Do your research before trying yohimbe, licorice root, or other potent herbs.

Grinding Herbs

Grinding tougher roots, barks, and mushrooms into powders before brewing releases their beneficial compounds. Use a dedicated coffee/spice grinder or mortar and pestle. Work in small batches to avoid overheating. Store freshly ground powders in sealed jars out of sunlight.

Most leaves and petals can simply be torn or cut. Avoid grinding gentler herbs like spearmint or chamomile which quickly release volatile essential oils when cut or crushed. Grind only firmer roots, rhizomes, barks, and dried mushrooms.

Boosting Bioavailability

Bioavailability refers to how readily an herb's nutrients and phytochemicals get absorbed and utilized by your body. Using fats, spices, and acids when preparing herbal tea can enhance bioavailability. Add lemon, ACV, ginger, piperine, and coconut milk to teas.

However, avoid diluting potency when seeking to concentrate benefits in a small volume of tea. Steep herbs fully before adding bioavailability-boosting ingredients. Foods containing fats taken alongside tea can amp absorption without diluting infused compounds.

Herbal Tea Recommendations

If you are new to drinking herbal teas medicinally, start slowly with more gentle everyday nourishment brews like tulsi, chamomile, rooibos, honeybush, lemon balm, and mint. Try adding these into your routine first before incorporating more potent herbs.

Target herbal teas toward your most pressing health goals or concerns. Refer back to the recipes and profiles throughout this chapter. For example, focus on prostate and urinary flow teas for BPH symptoms or ashwagandha and mucuna teas for low testosterone.

Be patient and allow at least 2-4 weeks of daily consumption to notice the benefits of teas like Tribulus for libido, ashwagandha for cortisol, holy basil for anxiety or fo-ti for healthy aging. The cumulative effects build gradually with routine use.

Pay attention to how your body responds to new herbs as your guide for which become staples. Notice if certain teas make you feel overstimulated or agitated. Avoid any that disrupt your sleep. However, short-term discomfort may indicate a detox process.

Herbal Tea Journey

Adding even one cup of herbal medicinal tea to your daily routine provides incremental benefits that compound over time. Let your exploration of the vast world of herbal teas as medicine be an ongoing journey. Keep expanding your knowledge and experiments.

Use the recipes, profiles, and tips in this chapter as a launching point for your herbal tea discovery. Tailor your daily brews to address your personal health goals while exploring new-to-you botanicals. Keep detailed notes on your experiences.

Herbal teas can fully replace daily caffeine, soda, or energy drink habits for clean hydration and nourishment. Allow yourself to make mistakes and learn from overstepping or using herbs that don't agree with you. Play and have fun!

Growing a windowsill herb garden provides the ultimate fresh tea ingredients. Even just having an aloe vera plant and spearmint on your kitchen counter ensures you can harvest components for nightly cups of tea. Get acquainted with nearby nurseries that carry a wide selection of potted medicinal herbs.

Commit to memory 5-10 herbs that serve as staples you consistently keep stocked in your kitchen to mix and match. For example, ashwagandha, Shatavari, brahmi, fennel seed, hibiscus, passionflower, and cassia cinnamon may become your herbal arsenal. Supplement with new seasonal herbs.

Let your herbal tea practice grow and evolve over your lifetime. As you age, teas that provide hormone balance, mental acuity, urinary flow help, inflammation relief, and restorative sleep promotion will only become more valuable. Herbal teas are the medicine you can enjoy daily!

More Herbal Teas for Men's Health

While we've covered an extensive array of beneficial herbs for men's health in tea form so far in this chapter, there are still many more botanicals to discover. The world of herbal tea formulations is truly vast and can be continually expanded over a lifetime.

Let's explore 20 more healing herbs for targeting common men's complaints like inflammation, stress, poor sleep, mental fog, sluggish digestion, skin conditions, aches, and pains. Gather inspiration for continuing to craft your own custom daily herbal tea rituals.

Herbal Tea for Inflammation
Chronic inflammation underlies many disease processes and accelerated aging. Countering systemic inflammation helps relieve

joint pain, gut issues, skin conditions, and vulnerability to illness. Anti-inflammatory herbs in tea provide healing benefits without side effects.

Turmeric contains the powerful compound curcumin to systematically reduce inflammatory prostaglandins and cytokines. Turmeric also enhances detoxification and provides antioxidant protection. Add fresh turmeric root or powdered tea daily.

Ginger root has been used for thousands of years in Traditional Chinese and Ayurvedic medicine for its warming anti-inflammatory effects. Gingerol blocks pain signaling while reducing swelling. Fresh ginger energizes tea while calming nausea, cramps, and arthritic pain.

Green tea possesses anti-inflammatory polyphenols like EGCG that inhibit the activity of pro-inflammatory molecules like NF-kB. Powerful antioxidants called catechins also defend against oxidative damage driving chronic inflammation.

Herbal Tea for Stress

Chronic stress keeps the body in a constant state of elevated cortisol which suppresses immunity, digestion, libido, sleep, and cognition. Adaptogenic herbs counteract the effects of prolonged stress when taken routinely.

Ashwagandha, as discussed earlier in this chapter, is one of the most powerful Ayurvedic adaptogens for lowering elevated cortisol and regulating neurotransmitters involved in the stress response like GABA. Daily ashwagandha promotes calm and hormonal balance.

Holy basil, also called tulsi, provides mentally uplifting yet physically relaxing effects. The concentrated source of antioxidants, triterpenes, and flavonoids in tulsi tea enhances the health of the mind, body, and emotions. Tulsi fortifies adaptogenic resilience.

Rhodiola rosea concentrates compounds called rosavins that help the body adapt to all types of stressors including fatigue, anxiety, exhaustion, environmental pollution, radiation, illness, and depression. Rhodiola boosts energy, mental performance, and stamina.

Herbal Tea for Restorative Sleep

Quality sleep is foundational to hormones, metabolism, brain health, immunity, and vitality. Certain nervine herbs promote relaxation while addressing causes of restlessness like anxiety, insomnia, muscle tension, and indigestion that disrupt sleep rhythms.

Chamomile is one of the most widely used herbs for promoting sleep due to its mild sedative properties. The aromatic volatile oils in chamomile tea bind to GABA receptors to instill a tranquilizing effect that relaxes the mind and body.

Passionflower contains bioflavonoids called chrysin that impart muscle-relaxing, sedative, and anxiety-reducing effects. Drinking passionflower tea before bed significantly improves sleep quality and next-day function without morning brain fog.

Valerian root increases gamma-aminobutyric acid (GABA) activity to calm overactive nerves while also relaxing smooth muscle tissue. This soothing herb enables deeper, more restorative non-REM and REM sleep for those struggling with insomnia.

Chapter 11

Herbal Teas for Cold & Flu Relief

Getting sick with a cold or the flu can really disrupt your life. Between the sore throat, coughing, congestion, fever, and aches, you can feel completely miserable. During cold and flu season, we tend to reach for conventional over-the-counter medications to help provide symptom relief. However, sipping on medicinal herbal teas can provide a natural way to minimize your suffering and help you recover faster.

Many herbs have been used for centuries in traditional healing practices for their antiviral, antimicrobial, and anti-inflammatory properties. Drinking tea made from the right herbs can tackle cold and flu symptoms from multiple angles. Let's explore some of the top herbal teas to help you fight off these seasonal viruses.

Antiviral Herbal Teas
At the first sign of a scratchy throat or sniffles, brewing up antiviral herbal teas can help halt viruses in their tracks. Some of the best antiviral herbs to combat colds and flu include elderberry, echinacea, oregano, rosehip, licorice root, ginger, and garlic.

Elderberry in particular has gained popularity in recent years for its stellar antiviral and immune-boosting abilities. The deep purple berries contain high levels of antioxidants called anthocyanins.

These compounds have potent anti-inflammatory and antiviral effects. Research indicates that elderberries can help reduce flu duration by several days. It works by blocking viruses from penetrating cells and replicating. Sipping elderberry tea at the onset of illness can help stop viruses dead in their tracks.

Echinacea is another heavy-hitting antiviral herb to incorporate into tea blends. Traditional herbalists have relied on echinacea for centuries to treat colds and upper respiratory infections. Modern research confirms its ability to enhance the immune system. Studies show echinacea ramps up the production of infection-fighting white blood cells, along with antiviral proteins like interferon. The three most commonly used species are E. purpurea, E. pallida, and E. angustifolia.

Oregano also displays powerful antiviral capabilities, thanks to compounds like thymol, carvacrol, and rosmarinic acid. These antimicrobial phenols found in oregano work against a wide variety of viruses and bacteria. Oregano makes a wonderful addition to herbal tea blends to stop illness right away. Just be sure to use Food-grade oregano oil, not the seasoning in your spice rack.

Rosehips are the fruit of the rose plant and are incredibly high in vitamin C. Rosehip tea delivers this immune-boosting vitamin along with antioxidants like carotenoids and bioflavonoids. Together, these nutrients block viruses from attaching and penetrating cells. Sipping rosehip tea can help prevent and shorten the duration of colds and flu.

Licorice root contains antiviral components like glycyrrhizic acid that prevent viruses from replicating. It also acts as an expectorant and cough suppressant. Licorice has a very sweet flavor that makes a nice complement to other herbs in tea blends. Those with certain medical conditions should avoid licorice root.

Ginger's warming heat and zing come from gingerols that display antiviral effects against respiratory viruses. Ginger also reduces inflammation and pain associated with illness. Fresh ginger root makes an energizing, spicy addition to herbal teas.

Fever Reducer: Boneset, Feverfew, and Yarrow Tea

When you're knocked flat on your back with the chills, body aches, and high fever that often accompany a bad cold or flu, getting some relief from your misery is a priority. While fever serves the important purpose of creating an inhospitable environment for invading viruses and bacteria, excessively high temperatures leave you feeling drained and just plain awful.

Thankfully, nature provides some excellent herbal fever reducers that can gently guide your body temperature back down to a comfortable level. Sipping on a medicinal cup of tea blending herbs like boneset, feverfew, and yarrow is a tasty way to minimize feverish discomfort so you can get back on your feet again.

Dating all the way back to traditional Cherokee medicine, boneset has a long history of use for alleviating fever. In the early 1800s, boneset earned a reputation as a cure-all remedy, with many people believing it could literally "break" fevers. The herb's healing abilities come from antimicrobial quinones as well as anti-inflammatory flavonoids like kaempferol, rutin, and quercetin.

Beyond just reducing high temperatures, boneset provides the added benefit of relieving the deep muscle aches and joint pains that often accompany fever. Sipping boneset tea can safely lower elevated body heat while also easing general discomfort. It helps fight off the underlying microbial infection as well.

Joining forces in this herbal fever-fighting trio is feverfew. Sometimes called "medieval aspirin," feverfew has been used since ancient Greek and Roman times for lowering high fevers and easing other related symptoms like headaches. The flowers and leaves of feverfew contain a compound called parthenolide that helps dilate constricted blood vessels in the brain that can trigger migraines.

In addition to parthenolide, feverfew contains potent anti-inflammatory substances like tanetin and aryl naphthalene. Together, these medicinal components provide cooling, soothing relief from the misery of high temperatures and associated body aches, headaches, or other discomforts.

Yarrow rounds out the natural fever reducers, providing a sweetly bitter medicinal tea. Traditional use of yarrow dates back to Ancient Greece and Rome for treating fevers and other ailments. The flavonoids in yarrow contain salicylic acid, giving this flowering herb pain-relieving abilities similar to aspirin.

Sore Throat Soother: Licorice Root, Marshmallow Root and Slippery Elm Tea

That sore, scratchy, irritated sensation in the back of your throat is one of the most annoying symptoms that accompanies a bad cold or flu. Caused by swollen tissues and inflammation, sore throats make it painful to swallow even liquids or your own saliva. The natural reaction is to avoid eating or drinking anything, which quickly leads to dehydration and further misery.

Thankfully, brewing up a medicinal cup or two of tea blending licorice root, marshmallow root, and slippery elm can provide sweet, soothing relief from throat discomfort. Sipping this herbal infusion coats and protects your throat while also tackling the root causes of irritation and inflammation. Before you know it, you'll be back to pain-free eating and drinking.

Licorice root, with its distinctive sweet flavor, has an impressive resume when it comes to taming sore throat misery. Containing beneficial compounds like glycyrrhizic acid, licorice exhibits antiviral, antimicrobial, and anti-inflammatory effects - the perfect triple threat for irritated throats. Sipping licorice root tea can destroy the bacteria or viruses provoking throat inflammation in the first place, while also easing swelling and discomfort.

Marshmallow root makes an ideal partner, providing extra mucilaginous soothing power. The high concentration of polysaccharides in marshmallow forms a slick, protective layer over mucous membranes in the throat when brewed as a tea. Studies show marshmallow root can effectively reduce throat pain and discomfort. At the same time, it thins out mucus secretions to make coughs more productive.

Rounding out this dynamic sore throat-soothing trio is slippery elm. True to its name, slippery elm bark contains abundant mucilage that transforms into a gel when mixed with water, coating and protecting irritated tissues. Slippery elm is one of the herbs most renowned for alleviating throat inflammation and rawness, allowing for comfortable swallowing.

Chest and Sinus Opener: Peppermint, Eucalyptus, Oregano Tea

That miserable, mucus-filled sensation deep in your head and chest is all too familiar when you're down with a cold or flu. Stuffy sinuses make it hard to breathe through your nose, while chest congestion leads to disruptive coughing fits as you try in vain to clear out the gunk filling your airways. This respiratory misery certainly takes a toll, making rest and recovery difficult.

Thankfully, brewing up a steamy cup of aromatic herbs like peppermint, eucalyptus and oregano can provide some relief for chest and sinus congestion. These herbs contain powerful compounds that work together to open up your airways, thin out mucus, fight infection, and help you breathe easier again.

Peppermint, with its distinctive crisp, cooling flavor, is one of the most widely used herbs for alleviating congestion and draining clogged sinuses. Peppermint contains a volatile oil called menthol that thins out mucus secretions so they don't sit thick and stagnant in respiratory tracts. Menthol also acts as a decongestant and cough suppressant, relaxing inflamed airways.

Beyond clearing congestion, peppermint exhibits impressive antimicrobial effects against viruses that cause respiratory infections like colds and flus. Sipping peppermint tea can tackle illness while opening up your nasal passages and chest for clearer breathing. Try adding a few sprigs of fresh peppermint to your cup for an extra dose of decongesting compounds.

Another aromatic herb renowned for treating chest congestion is eucalyptus. Eucalyptus contains a powerful compound called cineole that decreases mucus secretion in the lungs and acts as an expectorant to loosen phlegm. Cineole's vapor action helps clear nasal passages as well.

Cough Suppressant: Thyme, Plantain Leaf, Coltsfoot Tea

Dry, nagging coughs are one of the most annoying and disruptive symptoms that tend to linger endlessly when you're battling a cold or flu. The ceaseless coughing seems impossible to control, leaving your throat raw and keeping you up at night unable to rest. While coughing serves the important purpose of clearing mucus, germs, or other irritants from your airways, excessive coughing quickly becomes its own form of misery.

Thankfully, nature provides us with some excellent herbal cough suppressants. Sipping on a soothing cup of tea blending demulcent, expectorant, and antispasmodic herbs like thyme, plantain leaf, and coltsfoot can calm coughing fits. This allows you to get the restorative rest you need to recover, while still being able to clear your airways productively. Let's explore how these remarkable cough-taming herbs can work together to minimize your suffering.

Thyme's comforting, savory flavor comes from its abundance of volatile oils, flavonoids, and antioxidant phenolic acids. One key compound called thymol exhibits an antitussive effect, reducing coughing spasms and sensitivity in the throat and lungs. Thyme relaxes the bronchial tubes to minimize coughing fits. It also tackles bacterial or viral infections that may be provoking disruptive coughing in the first place.

Sipping some thyme tea can help take the edge off nagging coughs without completely suppressing your cough reflex. Thyme makes an excellent base for cough-calming herbal infusions. For best results, use about 1 teaspoon of fresh leaves or ½ teaspoon of dried thyme per cup of hot water, steeping for at least 5 minutes before drinking.

Plantain leaf perfectly complements thyme's soothing properties on irritating coughs. Studies demonstrate that the mucilage in plantain leaves helps coat and protect irritated mucous membranes in the throat and small airways. This slippery mucus soothes coughing while speeding healing.

Sniffle Stopper: Ginger, Lemon, Raw Honey, and Cayenne Tea

That dripping, constantly running nose, and stuffy head congestion are two of the most annoying symptoms that accompany a cold or flu. Excess mucus production leaves you sniffling and needing to blow your nose every few minutes.

Thankfully, several natural ingredients likely sitting in your kitchen right now can be combined into a dynamic tea to minimize those bothersome sniffles. Ginger, lemon, raw honey, and cayenne pepper make the perfect sniffle-stopping blend when brewed into a zesty medicinal beverage.

Ginger's warming heat and zing come from its abundance of active compounds called gingerols, shogaols, and zingerones. These spicy phenolic compounds exhibit antihistamine and decongestant effects, calming mucus hypersecretion and sneezing fits. Sipping ginger tea helps dry up excessive mucus production.

Ginger also contains potent antimicrobial and anti-inflammatory agents, like beta-bisabolene and zingiberene, that tackle viruses or bacteria provoking upper respiratory symptoms. Enjoying some fresh ginger tea can minimize congestion and post-nasal drip quickly and naturally. Use 1 inch of sliced fresh root per cup of hot water for best results.

Bright, lively lemon can also help combat cold and flu viruses while providing sinus-clearing benefits. Lemon is packed with immune-boosting vitamin C and antioxidants called limonoids that help thin out mucus. Squeezing in the juice from half a lemon into your tea delivers a refreshing citrus blast ideal for opening up stuffy nasal passages.

A dollop of local raw honey, with its sweet flavor and immune-enhancing properties, is another must for sniffle-fighting tea. Beekeepers recommend consuming honey sourced within 100 miles of where you live to help train your body's defenses against local allergens and illness. The enzymes and phytonutrients in raw honey give it antibacterial and wound-healing benefits as well.

closing remarks: And with that, we've reached the final page in our exploration of the remarkable world of herbal teas. What an incredible, flavorful, healing journey it's been!

Starting with the basics, we learned what makes herbal teas so special. Unlike traditional teas derived from the camellia sinensis plant, herbal teas can be made from the roots, seeds, flowers, fruits, and leaves of thousands of plants. This creates an incredibly diverse palette of flavors, colors, and health benefits unique to the herbs used.

We discussed the myriad wellness advantages herbal teas offer, from soothing stress to strengthening immunity. Their antioxidants, anti-inflammatories, and antimicrobials provide natural therapeutic actions for many conditions. Yet herbal teas are also simply a comforting, enjoyable beverage to savor daily.

Equipped with foundational knowledge, we explored brewing the perfect cup of herbal tea. From water temperature to steeping methods, proper preparation optimizes the flavor and medicinal compounds extracted into your cup. Don't underestimate the impact of these simple brewing techniques on your enjoyment of herbal tea.

The heart of our journey delved into herbal tea recipes organized by wellness needs, flavors, and individual herbs. We covered formulations for energy, digestion, immunity, relaxation, women's health, sleep, detoxing, and more. From chamomile vanilla sleep tea to dandelion detox blend, moringa energy brew to throat coat, each recipe enlightened us on new herbal ingredients.

Use this book as inspiration to create your own signature recipes based on your tastes and what your body needs. Become your own herbalist experimenting with new ingredient combinations. The only limit is your imagination.

As you continue enjoying herbal teas, remember to choose high-quality herbs from ethical sources. Handle herbs with care to preserve their potency. Remain ever curious and open to learning as science uncovers new benefits of medicinal plants.

Above all, let herbal teas be nourishing rituals that promote mindfulness, presence, stillness, and connection - with your body, the plants, and the moment. May herbal teas always be healing transformations, both physical and spiritual.

Thank you for joining me on this flavorful wellness journey! May it inspire you to brew your own cup of natural magic every day. Here's to the power of plants bringing health into your life, one tea at a time. Go out and sip your way to well-being!